STEVEN G. ALDANA, PH.D.

The
Culprit

&The
Cure

**Why *lifestyle* is the culprit
behind America's poor health** / **and how *transforming* that
lifestyle can be the cure**

MAPLE
MOUNTAIN
PRESS

MAPLETON, UTAH

Visit us at www.maplemountainpress.com or call toll free (866) 732-3843

Library of Congress Cataloging-in-Publication Data

Aldana, Steven G., 1962-
    The culprit and the cure: how lifestyle is the culprit behind America's poor
    health and how transforming that lifestyle can be the cure / Steven G. Aldana.
    p. cm.
    Includes bibliographical references and index.
    LCCN 2004111912
    ISBN 0-9758828-0-5

    1. Health behavior--United States. 2. Chronic diseases--United States--Prevention.
    3. Behavior modification--United States. I. Title.

RA776.9.A43 2005   613'.0973
                        QBI04-200466

Printed in the United States of America
Phoenix Color Corp., Hagerstown, MD

Layout design and art direction by Bjorn W. Pendleton
Pendleton Creative, LLC | www.pendletoncreative.com

Contents

Preface

I WAS ONE OF THOSE STRANGE YOUNG MEN who actually liked school. I graduated from college with a degree in physical education and minors in mathematics and geology. I thought I was really learning a lot when I got my master's and doctorate degrees and then took a job teaching and doing research at a university. Because of my research activities, I was frequently in hospitals to make sure our research procedures were being followed correctly. Between observing procedures and gathering research data, I was able to walk the halls of several hospitals around the country and visit with a variety of physicians.

Seeing all of these patients come and go, I couldn't help but wonder, "Where do they all come from? What caused them to have chronic diseases that were so bad that they needed extensive medical procedures?" It seemed there was no end to the constant supply of new patients coming to hospitals for medical treatment. I recall listening to cardiologists, surgeons, and other physicians complain that they felt almost powerless to stop the tide of chronic diseases they were seeing every day.

My research and teaching experiences caused me to seriously question what I had learned in school and gave me the motivation I needed to further explore the true causes of most of the poor health we all see and experience. After twelve years of teaching and researching, I took a sabbatical leave to refine my skills and become exposed to new ways of thinking.

Rather than move to some exotic destination and experience peace and tranquility abroad, I did something most professors would not consider: I stayed home, in my office. I read just about every scientific article ever published on nutrition, physical activity, and chronic diseases. I searched for articles in journals, got copies of them, and spent hours, days, and even weeks reading, comparing, summarizing, and questioning all of them. If I came across a topic I did not understand, I took a break and read other materials until I knew what I was reading and could understand everything the researchers had done.

Until my sabbatical, I thought I was well educated and that I had a very good understanding of what a healthy lifestyle is. I had even considered myself an expert on good health. In reality, my understanding was woefully incomplete.

What I learned during my sabbatical changed my life; it changed my perspective; it changed the way I thought about health. It was as if, for the first time, I really understood what I was supposed to do with my life. What I had learned had such a powerful effect on me that I knew I needed to organize my thoughts and ideas—which was the start of this book.

I can summarize all of this learning in two sentences: Most of the chronic diseases and deaths in Westernized societies are not caused by genetics or some act of God. They are the direct result of poor nutrition, lack of physical activity, and tobacco use.

The most frightening part of my experience is that my new knowledge and perspective put me directly in the center of no-man's-land. Let me explain. In the world there are exercise scientists who know everything about exercise, nutritionists who know a lot about nutrition, and behavioral psychologists who know a lot about helping people change behaviors. Rarely do these three professions interact with each other. They are content to work in their own worlds, sometimes oblivious to what the others are doing because of an attitude of "they are not one of us."

At one university where I taught, a new course was being created to help students learn how to have a healthy lifestyle. The exercise science faculty felt the course should include just fitness concepts, the nutritionists believed the course should focus on good nutrition, and the behavioral psychologists weren't even invited to the meetings. No one in the meetings understood the importance of all three pieces.

If you want to have a long, healthy life, you need to adopt a healthy diet (nutrition) and be regularly physically active (exercise), and you need to maintain those behaviors (psychology) for the rest of your life. The committee members all had tunnel vision and could not accept opinions or positions that were outside their traditional belief systems. There are a few nutritionists, exercise experts, and psychologists who understand this, but not nearly as many as there should be.

This no-man's-land extends deep into the medical profession. Physicians are traditionally trained to treat disease, and they do an excellent job of helping people get back on their feet when disease occurs. However, our current health care system is not a health care system at all. It is a disease care system—and an excellent one at that.

Have you ever gone to see your physician when you were feeling fine and just wanted more advice on what you could do to continue feeling fine? Not likely. Physicians receive virtually no training on nutrition or physical activity in medical school. How could they, when there is already an enormous amount of information and skills they have to learn in a very short amount of time?

Besides, in no-man's-land, insurance companies don't pay a physician to talk to you about nutrition and physical activity. Insurance companies pay for procedures, medications, and treatments, but give little more than lip service to healthy behavior change. There is no money for those physicians who practice prevention. Unless a physician takes time to educate patients about the importance of a healthy lifestyle—and a few do—patients are not going to get much advice about prevention. Hopefully this will change.

County health departments offer vaccinations, lactation programs, HIV testing, and other traditional community health practices. Just like physicians, however, they are generally out of their element when asked to teach patients about good nutrition, physical activity, and healthy lifestyle behaviors. In no-man's-land, few want to or know how to practice disease prevention.

In one of the most bizarre twists of our capitalist society, worksites, not medical professionals, have played the largest role in helping people have healthy lifestyles. That's right, the only group to rally behind the need to improve lifestyles is employers. Manufacturers, retail establishments, service industries, transportation industries, municipalities, and most other employment sectors provide not only jobs, benefits, and needed services, they also provide health-promotion programs for employees. They are actively involved in the promotion of healthy lifestyles.

Some employers believe this is the right thing to do for employees because individuals are their most valuable assets. Most others, however, do it because it is expensive to have an unhealthy workforce. In 2003, health care costs for companies across the United States increased an average of 14%.[1] The yearly premiums for employer-sponsored health plans rose to $3,383 for single coverage and $9,068 for family coverage. Companies know that if they can help their employees adopt healthy lifestyles, the employees will have less chronic diseases, be absent less, and have fewer health care costs. It is truly a strange society we live in when health care becomes the responsibility of individual employers, corporations, and companies—yet that is precisely the situation. Worksites with health-promotion programs are boldly moving into no-man's-land. If you work for an employer that has a health-promotion program, you may get some help in your quest for good health.

A few federal agencies, like the Centers for Disease Control and Prevention and the Healthier US initiative from Health and Human Services, are also taking responsibility for promoting healthy lifestyles. Most likely you have heard of the 5-a-day campaign used to promote consumption of more fruits and vegetables. However, with the exception of these and a few other programs, you are on your own. You are left with your own survival instinct to try to find the truth in a sea of marketing propaganda, aggressive advertising, media spin, outright lies, and just plain ignorance.

The fourteen chapters of this book are divided into three parts. They are the why, what, and how of healthy living. Part I explains why a healthy lifestyle can do more to improve your health than any other single medical breakthrough of the past 100 years. In Part II you will learn what is required for good nutrition and regular physical activity. The best information is found in Part III—how to change your eating and exercise behaviors for life, and how to attain a healthy body weight along the way.

The information presented in these chapters is not my opinion. It is not a collection of health tips I've picked up from friends and relatives. This information comes directly from the best researchers and scientists in the world whose findings have been published only after their research has been carefully scrutinized by other nationally and internationally known experts. This information is the most accurate information available to date, and it has the potential to change your life. If there are any errors in the book, they are my own and I take full responsibility for them.

A good friend sent me a family photo taken at Niagara Falls. The amount of water tumbling over that cliff is awesome. It reminded me of our nation's current health situation. I imagined thousands of people floating in the river above the falls. Most of them were swept over the falls, where teams of medical professionals treated their injuries and tried to help them recover. Upstream I imagined someone standing on the bank throwing out a lifeline to anyone who wanted to grab hold and be pulled ashore to a warm, dry, safe place.

This book is your lifeline. Grab hold of it, read it carefully, and use it to adopt a healthy lifestyle. If you do, you will likely increase your lifespan, improve the quality of your life, and dramatically improve your health. And with time, no-man's-land will become a healthy, vibrant metropolitan community.

1.   Kaiser Family Foundation/Health Research and Educational Trust. 2003 Annual Employer Benefits Survey. Menlo Park, CA; 2003. Available at: http://www.kff.org/statepolicy/chp031604pkg.cfm

Acknowledgments

It is easy to write a book on health when you surround yourself with people who are smarter, better organized, and even healthier than you are.

I want to thank Doctors Roger Greenlaw, Hans Diehl, Walter Willett, David Hunnicutt, Troy Adams, Nico Pronk, John Kelly, and Ron Goetzel. Tim Butler, David Koehler, Aaron Hardy, Bill Whitmer, Garry Lindsay, Lisa Henning, and Lynne Nilson also provided valuable reviews of earlier drafts. Dean Robert Conlee has always supported my efforts to make the best science available to the public, despite opposition from other academics and peers, and I wish to thank him for that support.

No one knows my writing weaknesses more than my secretary, Maggie Shibla. I credit her with turning my manuscript drafts into something of value. Her insights, corrections, and real-world sense were just what I needed to keep this book focused on you, the American public.

Bjorn Pendleton is a book-designing genius.

I wish to thank Laura Rawlins and her team of copy editors, who did a wonderful job of polishing the final manuscript.

I want to thank the people at the National Library of Medicine, who had the foresight to put all of the 14 million science articles in one searchable database—PubMed. Without this service it would not have been possible for me to find, copy, read, and summarize hundreds of research articles.

My wife, Diana, and each of my wonderful children have allowed me the time and energy to focus my passion and write this book.

Lastly, my abilities to analyze, write, learn, and conduct research are not something I developed on my own. For reasons I don't fully understand, I have always been a curious, probing, and inquisitive being. I was born that way. Nothing I did as a child could have given me these abilities. This and other experiences in my life suggest to me that there must be a supreme being controlling our universe. My heart tells me this is true. To a patient, loving, and mysterious God, I give thanks.

PART ONE

Why

Introduction

We cannot become what we need to be
by remaining what we are.
—Max De Pree

IN THE PAST FEW DECADES, the amount of scientific information available on the importance of regular physical activity and good nutrition has grown dramatically. This information has helped researchers better understand how a healthy diet and regular exercise affect disease processes and what benefits are available to those who have a healthy lifestyle. Each day new research findings are reported in scientific journals, conferences, and press releases. As new information is produced, it is added to what is already known, and the entire collection of findings is reevaluated and critiqued in an effort to determine the best ways to live our lives. Unfortunately, there is a huge gap between what is known scientifically about eating healthy and exercising and what most citizens of the United States and other Westernized countries actually do.

For example, we now know that approximately 40% of all cancers are caused by the typical American diet, lack of physical activity, and obesity, and that cancer is mostly a preventable disease.[1] Research has shown that if individuals eat five servings of fruits and vegetables per day, the chance of getting several cancers can be dramatically reduced.[2] Despite this information, only 20% of Americans consume five servings of fruits and vegetables a day.[3] Also, most Americans fail to get enough physical activity to receive any health benefits.[4] In order to extend life, improve the quality of life, and avoid the onset of chronic diseases, the gap between what is currently known and what Americans actually do needs to be reduced.

What We Know

We all suffer from the normal short-term bumps, bruises, and illnesses of life, but when asked to name illnesses or conditions that last for many years, are persistent, and eventually lead to death, most people list cancer, heart disease, stroke, arthritis, Alzheimer's disease, and diabetes. These diseases are called *chronic diseases* and are responsible for seven out of every ten deaths in the United States. Chronic diseases are among the most common and costly health problems to treat, but they are also among the most preventable.

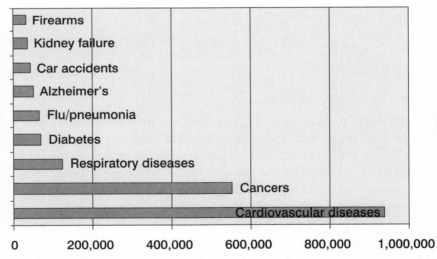

Figure 1.1 Leading causes of death in the United States, 2002

Chronic diseases don't just happen; they are almost entirely the result of decades of unhealthy living. This means children, teenagers, young adults, and seniors who eat a typical American diet and don't exercise regularly are developing chronic diseases such as diabetes and heart disease and are increasing their risk of getting cancer. It is scary to think that children might be developing heart disease, but that is precisely what is happening (more on this later).

If a person has a healthy diet, does not smoke, and exercises regularly, the odds of that person getting one of these diseases are much lower. While a healthy lifestyle isn't a guarantee that you won't become chronically ill, it does tilt the odds heavily in your favor.

Figure 1.2 shows results from a variety of studies that have evaluated the relationships between healthy lifestyle and several chronic diseases. The bars indicate the percentage of all cases of the diseases listed that could be prevented. Let's put this into perspective. Each year in the United States, over 700,000 people die of heart disease. According to the research reported in this figure, 82% of these deaths—560,000 deaths per year—are caused by lack of exercise, poor diet, and tobacco use. If we apply the same calculations to other chronic diseases, over 1.6 million deaths in the United States could potentially be avoided every year.

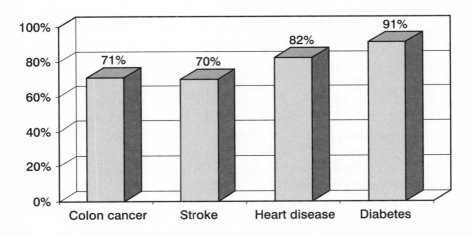

Figure 1.2 Percent of selected chronic diseases that are avoidable[5-7]

Some might say that if you prevent chronic diseases, you prevent death, and if you prevent death, you live forever. Well, no one is claiming to have a surefire way to avoid the Grim Reaper, and preventing chronic diseases does not mean preventing death. But preventing chronic disease does mean you can determine, in large measure, how and when you will die. In fact, more than likely, you have already done this: Have you ever taken an antibiotic? Have you ever been in a car accident while wearing a seatbelt? Have you ever been vaccinated or had surgery? If you have, you have most likely delayed the time of your death.

The exact impact of healthy living on life span is not known, but several studies have provided some fairly accurate estimates. For example, let's assume that you decide to eat nuts five times a week. Would that affect how long you live? A review of all studies on this topic show that, on average, you would gain almost three years of life compared to those who rarely eat nuts. Similar studies have been completed on other risks:[8,9]

People who	Live an extra
Are vegetarian	1.5 years
Exercise regularly	2.4 years
Eat nuts five times a week	2.5 years
Have normal blood pressure	3.7 years
Are not diabetic	6.6 years
Maintain normal weight	11 years

The differences in life span shown here are independent of each other, meaning that if you changed just one part of your life, like exercise, there is an increase in the life span associated with that one change. What happens if you change several aspects of your lifestyle? Let's assume someone exercises regularly (2.4 years), eats plenty of nuts (2.5 years), and has normal blood pressure (3.7 years). What could happen to his or her life span? One could roughly estimate that the total years saved by these health factors equals 8.6 years (2.4 + 2.5 + 3.7 = 8.6 years).

Now, these calculations are not exact and cannot be used to determine additional years of life for any one individual. But for a large group of people who adopt these behaviors, the average increase in life span would be around 8.6 years. And while these additional years don't tell us how many years life will be extended, they do tell us that if we were to compare the life spans of a group of people who maintained this lifestyle with a group who did not, the difference between their life spans would be around 8.6 years.

There are several populations located in the United States that demonstrate that a healthy lifestyle does directly impact life span. Seventh-Day Adventists are encouraged to be vegetarians, and many members of this faith-based community abstain completely from consuming meat. Longitudinal studies of these vegetarians revealed that men in this group lived 7.3 years longer than the national average and the women lived 4.4 years longer. Those who also exercised, avoided tobacco use, and maintained a healthy body weight lived 10 years longer than average.[8]

Mormons in the state of California who exercised regularly, did not smoke, and got adequate sleep had death rates due to cancer and cardiovascular disease that were 70–80% lower than the rest of the nation. Males in this population lived an average of 11 years longer than comparable U.S. males, and females lived 7 years longer. By avoiding tobacco use, exercising regularly, and getting enough sleep, these Mormons demonstrated some of the lowest death rates ever published.[10] There is no doubt that if they had a healthy diet and maintained a healthy weight, the extensions of life they experienced could have been even greater, but at this time, there is no good data to predict how long life could really be.

What about Genetics?

Some chronic diseases are not lifestyle related. These are generally caused by an inherited genetic mutation or a toxic environment. Genes certainly play a role in the disease process, but that role is much smaller than you might believe.[11] Within some families, a gene that causes cancer or heart disease at an early age may be passed from generation to generation. These particularly aggressive genes can affect many members of a single family line and, though they almost always cause disease, they are rare—less than 5% of all cases of cancer and cardiovascular disease fall into this category. Other genes, which are not quite as aggressive, can also cause these diseases, but just carrying the gene doesn't mean you will develop the disease.

These weaker genes, called *polymorphisms,* can cause health problems only if they have the right environment. If you were a polymorphism and you wanted to develop into a disease, you would want to live in someone who ate a typical American diet, didn't exercise much, and smoked because this type of lifestyle would create an environment within the body that encourages unhealthy genes. On the other hand, when these less aggressive genes are surrounded by a diet of fruits, vegetables, and whole grains, they have difficulty reproducing successfully and cannot cause life-threatening conditions. Therefore, just because you inherit a gene that is known to cause problems doesn't mean you are destined to have those problems. Most genes can express themselves only if they have the right environment.

Living Well to the Very End

There are more benefits from living healthy than simply preventing chronic diseases and postponing death. The type of life you live is just as important as how long you live. Many researchers study factors that contribute to the value and meaning of life as well as people's happiness and contentment. These factors refer to a person's quality of life. Besides avoiding chronic diseases, people who have a healthy lifestyle often report having more energy, feeling more productive, having less stress, and being able to cope better with the demands and trials of everyday life. Additionally, they are able to maintain a healthy body weight and to enjoy all the social, physical, and psychological benefits that come from not being overweight or obese. One of the most important benefits of living well is the improvement of quality of life that occurs in later years.

Every year the average life span in the United States increases; Americans now live to an average age of 76 years. Those who adopt a healthy lifestyle live much longer than this. But what kind of quality of life do these extra years provide? No one wants a long life that is full of chronic illness, disability, or years of intensive, full-time nursing care.

At some point in the later years of life, most people experience a significant medical event. This could be a broken hip, a stroke, bypass surgery, or cancer. From that point until death, quality of life and the ability to function physically are dramatically reduced.[12] The amount of illness and limitations that often occur between these kinds of medical events and death are called "end-of-life poor health."[13] This unhealthy portion of life precedes death for many people, but research into the impact of living a healthy lifestyle on end-of-life morbidity tells us that there are even more benefits to healthy living.[14]

Individuals who eat right and exercise throughout their lives live longer. They still experience significant medical events toward the end of their lives, but, on average, the events are delayed between 7 and 13 years, and the time between the significant medical event and death is shortened.[15–16]

The term used to explain this is *compression of morbidity*. End-of-life poor health and dysfunction are reduced or compressed into a shorter amount of time. Major illness and significant physical and functional limitations still occur, but they don't seem to span as long a period of time, and they occur closer to the time of death. I like to joke that by living a healthy lifestyle, I plan to die at the age of 94 while skiing with my great-grandkids. I will probably hit a tree, suffer a significant medical event (fractured skull), slip into a coma (significant physical and functional limitation), and die that day. Now that's high-quality living and real compression of morbidity!

Realistically, those with a healthy lifestyle will live longer, suffer a serious medical event much later in life, and have a shorter period of time between the event and death. It's as if living a healthy lifestyle allows you to live a full, rich life well into old age, at which time you become ill, experience a rapid decline in health, and pass away. That sounds pretty appealing.

Extension and improvement of life is possible because of the avoidance of chronic diseases. By providing the body with the correct diet and exposing it regularly to the physiological and physical effects that come from regular exercise, the processes that lead to the onset of chronic diseases stop. This disease prevention occurs at the cellular level within the body.

In order to attain the most benefits from physical activity, all individuals should accumulate 30 minutes or more of moderate-intensity physical activity on most, preferably all, days of the week.

Even if you have not eaten well or exercised regularly in the past and chronic diseases processes have begun, you can still stop the progression—this suggests that it is never too late to change your lifestyle. Ideally these diseases should be prevented, but even if you have certain chronic diseases, a healthy lifestyle may be able to reverse the disease process and repair damaged tissues.[17–20]

Besides all of the medication and treatment options that are available, many physicians are realizing that a healthy lifestyle is important to prevent, arrest, and even reverse many chronic diseases. Some research has shown that a healthy diet and an active lifestyle can have a greater treatment effect than most of the common medications that doctors routinely prescribe.[21–23]

How to Live

So how can you be sure that what you are about to read is not another pitch from just another health expert who thinks he knows what is best for you and your health? I am only a messenger. Though I have published many of my own scientific papers showing the benefits of a healthy lifestyle, the information presented here is an up-to-date summary of the best information that is currently available. This information comes from the best scientists and researchers worldwide who have devoted their lives to understanding how to achieve good health. If you reject this information, you reject the advice from the brightest and wisest minds in the world.

Every day new research on diet and exercise is reported at scientific meetings or published in scientific journals. Sometimes this new information fits nicely with previously discovered concepts, but, unfortunately, research sometimes produces results that force us to think in ways that may not completely match what was previously thought. This is why recommendations for physical activity and good nutrition are updated and refined constantly.

The following recommendations for physical activity and nutrition are simple to understand and follow. This book is designed to help you understand why the current recommendations are accurate and vital to good health. Be warned that in the years to come, more information will be gathered that will force even these recommendations to be adjusted, but I wouldn't expect any drastic changes.

Hundreds of scientists and health professionals studied thousands of scientific results and concluded that in order to attain the most benefits from physical activity, *all individuals should accumulate 30 minutes or more of moderate-intensity physical activity on most, preferably all, days of the week.* This is it—decades of research, hundreds of millions of research dollars, all condensed into one simple statement.[24]

This statement does not reveal how a sedentary lifestyle can lead to premature death and disease, nor does it describe what happens to your body when you do exercise. This information is found in subsequent chapters. This physical activity recommendation seems simple, but few people follow it because in today's society it is difficult to stay physically active. That's why several chapters of this book are devoted to helping you adopt a physically active lifestyle and maintain regular activity for the rest of your life.

What should you eat to enjoy good health benefits? Thousands of research studies are summarized in the Healthy Eating Pyramid on the next page.[25] This pyramid is different from the Food Guide Pyramid you already know because it is based on the most current and complete scientific literature. It is not influenced by any dairy, meat, produce, or any other group with a vested interest in seeing a particular food displayed more prominently on the pyramid; it is based entirely on science.

You'll notice that this Healthy Eating Pyramid starts with a foundation of physical activity and healthy body weight. These are placed at the bottom because they are of critical importance to good health. Perhaps the most

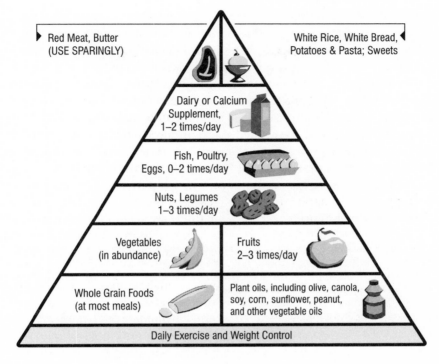

Red Meat, Butter
(USE SPARINGLY)

White Rice, White Bread,
Potatoes & Pasta; Sweets

Dairy or Calcium
Supplement,
1–2 times/day

Fish, Poultry,
Eggs, 0–2 times/day

Nuts, Legumes
1–3 times/day

Vegetables
(in abundance)

Fruits
2–3 times/day

Whole Grain Foods
(at most meals)

Plant oils, including olive, canola,
soy, corn, sunflower, peanut,
and other vegetable oils

Daily Exercise and Weight Control

Figure 1.3 Healthy Eating Pyramid. Adapted from www.hsph.harvard.edu/nutritionsource

notable impression this pyramid gives is that the healthiest foods are generally foods in their natural form—without heavy processing or alteration.

I'm keenly aware that some of you are looking at this recommendation and are rapidly entering a state of shock. Your current diet may look nothing like this, and you have no desire to change it. I sympathize with you and appeal to your sense of fairness. If after reading the rest of the evidence presented in this book, you still have no desire to make even small changes in your diet, I respect your traditions and opinions and thank you for your attention.

Some see this pyramid and think, "I'm doing pretty good. Look at all the foods on that pyramid I already eat!" You will find the evidence that supports this type of diet is so compelling that it motivates you to do even better, and the better you do, the more benefits you will receive. This book contains tips and strategies you can use to help you make positive changes in your diet and physical activity that will improve your health.

How Are We Doing Now?

Throughout this book, the most current information regarding healthy lifestyles and chronic diseases is provided. But to understand the importance of this information, it is good to know what our country's current lifestyles are. Each year the federal government conducts national health surveys to assess the health status of the nation. The information from these surveys helps us see trends and identify areas where the public needs to be informed and educated about important health concerns. The organization responsible for these studies is the Centers for Disease Control, now called the Centers for Disease Control *and Prevention*, a name change that provides a hint as to how our national focus is changing.

Other resources

The Centers for Disease Control and Prevention have written an outstanding brochure on the power of prevention. When you are done reading this book and want to learn more about the power of prevention, I suggest you read the brochure. To get an online copy, go to:

http://www.cdc.gov/nccdphp/power_prevention/pdf/power_of_prevention.pdf

---

Let me throw out a few tidbits about common health risks, and you draw your own conclusions about our current health status in the United States:[4]

1 out of 4 adults smokes
1 out of 3 adults has high blood pressure
1 out of 3 adults has high blood cholesterol
2 out of 3 adults are overweight or obese
3 out of 4 adults fail to get enough exercise
4 out of 5 adults need to significantly improve their diets

Over the past 40 years, fewer people have taken up smoking, but levels of blood pressure, blood cholesterol, and exercise participation have remained relatively unchanged. Over that same period, the number of overweight American children has quadrupled—more than 15% of all grade-school children are overweight today; as people age, the problem gets much worse.[3] In 2002, 60% of all adults in the United States were overweight or obese.[26]

Having health risks is not the same as having chronic diseases, but these health risks are directly related to chronic disease processes, and chronic diseases lead to death. Heart disease, stroke, cancer, and diabetes are four of the top six causes of death and account for 64% of all deaths. Americans and citizens of Westernized nations who smoke, eat an American-like diet, and avoid physical activity are more likely to suffer and die from these primarily avoidable chronic diseases.

How Did We Get This Way?

Before the 1900s, the average American spent most of the hours in a day preparing meals and gathering, growing, harvesting, and preserving food. Animals and humans provided the labor required for daily subsistence. Physical labor was the norm, and the primary mode of transportation was walking. It was common for someone to walk for miles to communicate, transact business, or purchase supplies. The foods consumed were very close to their natural form because processing was unavailable or expensive. For example, flour used in most bread was whole wheat, not the bleached white flour so widely used today. Fruits, vegetables, grains, and cereals were the sources of most carbohydrates and fats consumed, and meat was eaten sparingly.[27-28]

There has been a drastic change in dietary and physical activity patterns in the past 100 years. Cars and public transportation have replaced walking as the dominant modes of travel. Physical labor is still the norm for some construction workers, farm laborers, and manufacturers, but many Americans, both young and old, spend much of the day sitting in chairs at work, school, or play. According to the 2000 U.S. census, half of all homes have computers and Internet access (and chairs to go with those computers). In addition to computer and video-game time, 26% of U.S. children watch four or more hours of television per day, and 67% watch at least two hours per day.[29]

Washing machines, garage door openers, golf carts, television remotes, microwave ovens, bread mixers, dishwashers, and escalators help us avoid activity. We work diligently to avoid this physical activity, and inventors have done a fabulous job of developing laborsaving devices that make our lives easier and leave us more leisure time. Chances are you drive around the parking lot of a store or office until you find the parking stall that is closest to the door you wish to enter. Generally speaking we work hard to avoid exertion. Machines, advances in technology, and societal changes have altered our lives to such an extent that the causes of death so common a century ago have been almost entirely replaced by diseases of affluence—chronic diseases associated with an unlimited supply of inexpensive food and little need for physical activity.

Some of the most evident changes in our society are in the types and amounts of foods we eat. We now enjoy a tremendous variety of food and are confident that most foods are safe and protected from toxins and bacteria. Virtually any food can be acquired at any time of the year. Compared to 100 years ago, today's diet consists of less fiber, fewer fruits and vegetables, and more meat, sugars, fats, and vitamins.[30-31]

Foods in their natural forms, such as fruits, vegetables, and whole grains, are still available, but the pressure to purchase processed, rich-tasting convenience foods is intense. In our free-market society, those who can produce, market, and sell foods that people want can influence public nutrition for better or worse. These marketing campaigns are extremely well funded, carefully targeted, and highly effective.

To see if any of these marketing campaigns have affected you, take the following quiz. Read the following corporate slogans and see if you can finish them by filling in the missing word or words. The answers are found in the box below.

1. You deserve a break today at _____.
2. Have it your way at _____.
3. Yo Quiero _____.
4. Everything's better with _____ on it.
5. _____ does a body good.
6. Finger lickin' _____.
7. Betcha can't eat just _____.
8. Breakfast of _____.
9. _____ melt in your mouth and not in your hand.
10. Snap! Crackle! _____
11. Sometimes you feel like a nut, _____.

ANSWERS: 1. McDonalds, 2. Burger King, 3. Taco Bell, 4. Blue Bonnet, 5. Milk, 6. good (KFC), 7. one (Lay's potato chips), 8. champions (Wheaties), 9. M&Ms, 10. Pop! (Kellogg's Rice Krispies), 11. sometimes you don't (Peter Paul Mounds)

Isn't it amazing how we remember slogans for food products we may not even like? The effective marketing of food permeates nearly every aspect of our lives. We see food promoted everywhere—strategically stacked at checkout stands, beautifully depicted in newspaper ads, cleverly incorporated into television shows, and marketed in radio ads. Pervasive morning television commercials specifically target children by advertising foods high in sugar and low in nutritional value.

A daily news and current events program called Channel One is viewed by 8.3 million school children every day. Schools pay nothing for the televisions or for installation or programming, but children must watch the program and the fast food commercials that support it. Virtually every school district receives lucrative contracts with food vendors if they agree to house vending machines. Visit any junior high or high school, and you see rows of vending machines promoting all sorts of yummy candies, soda, and high-fat foods children love to eat. Who can resist?

Adults are targets of primetime television commercials displaying fabulous buffets, endless refills, juicy meats, and serving sizes easily sufficient for two (or more). Regardless of where you live in America, you are likely in an environment that encourages unhealthy eating and sedentary living from the cradle to the grave. In the past century, we have changed from a nation that used to "eat to live" to one that "lives to eat"; an unpleasant side effect of this change is the premature death of most Americans.

Some would say that as long as no one is being forced to consume unhealthy foods and individuals are free to choose, then the individual and not the producers of food should be blamed for the resulting obesity and chronic disease problems. However, our communities and environments are so inundated with food advertising and marketing that it is extremely difficult to eat healthy when healthy choices are not available and you are under tremendous marketing pressure to do just the opposite. When was the last time you saw a primetime television commercial promoting fresh fruits, vegetables, or whole grains?

Change Is Possible, But It Isn't Easy

If the benefits of a healthy lifestyle are so great, why don't more people eat right and exercise regularly? Eating and exercising are basic human behaviors. A behavior is nothing more than a human response to some stimulus. When we feel hungry, we eat. Eating is the response or behavior that results from the hunger stimulus. Since everyone has to eat, the real decision is in choosing what to eat. Local culture, money, taste, time, and availability of food all help us determine what to eat, and changing this decision-making process is difficult.

Some people don't change because they may not have had the opportunity to learn what a healthy diet consists of, how much exercise is enough, and how these two lifestyle choices are directly related to the causes of death, disease, and poor quality of life. Even if people know why they should live a healthy lifestyle, lack of motivation, time, social support, and the presence of environmental pressure to eat unhealthy foods and to be sedentary often overwhelm their ability to change.

Eating and exercising behaviors are not unlike our financial behaviors. Most working adults are under pressure to use all their current income for things that are important to them. Of all working adults, only 44% voluntarily participate in any form of retirement savings because other, more pressing needs require funds that might otherwise be saved.[32]

As working adults get closer to retirement age, the number of individuals who actively save for retirement increases dramatically. Retirement, like many chronic diseases, doesn't happen until later in life, but it must be planned for early in life if individuals want to adequately prepare for the future. For many people, changing the types of food they eat is difficult, getting regular exercise is even more difficult, and maintaining a healthy weight is a losing battle.

When confronted with the most current information on diet, exercise, and disease, most people will at least begin to think about their own lives and how they might start to live better, and thinking about making change is the first step. To get the benefits of a healthy lifestyle, new behaviors need to be adopted. To help you overcome the difficulty of changing behaviors, the last part of this book gives you the skills, ideas, and practical know-how to adopt healthy lifestyles and maintain them for life.

Often I am asked, "How long do I have to exercise and eat right?" This is a great question, which I usually answer with another question: "How long do you want the benefits?" The benefits come relatively quickly and last for as long as the healthy foods are eaten and physical activity is enjoyed.

One man who was attempting to adopt a healthy lifestyle concluded that it wasn't worth it because, if he followed this advice for 50 years, the time he spent exercising would add up to one year—about the amount of time his life would be extended. He figured it wouldn't be worth it because he would have to spend a year exercising to gain one year of extra life. He decided he'd rather be sedentary and die a year earlier.

This interesting analytical justification for not exercising is only partially accurate. Sure, a 20-year-old who exercises regularly will spend about one year in physical activity by the age of 70, but this does not result in the simple addition of one year of life with an accumulated year of exercise. The benefits of regular physical activity are much greater.

Individuals who are physically active have an average life span closer to three years longer than individuals who are sedentary. In addition, the quality of life enjoyed by active individuals is considerably better. It is difficult to imagine how spending time hiking, golfing, walking with friends, or working in the yard could be all that bad.

This book gives you the skills, ideas, and practical know-how to adopt healthy lifestyles and maintain them for life.

After hearing a lecture on the importance of living a healthy lifestyle, two participants came by my office. The first, a 20-year-old male college student, came in to complain that he was not interested in changing his diet or getting exercise because he felt great. He could eat whatever he wanted, live however he wanted, and he generally felt great all the time. He even gladly reported that his blood pressure was perfect, his cholesterol was low, and he didn't smoke.

Right then he didn't have any major health problems and most likely wouldn't for another 30 years. He was not convinced that he should do anything differently, especially if what he was currently doing was working fine. He finished by saying, "'If it ain't broke, don't fix it,' and even if I do have problems, I'll just have the doctor fix me up."

The second individual was a 58-year-old female who had raised a family and now lived at home with her husband. Like most people over age 50, she was by definition obese, had high blood pressure and high blood cholesterol, and was recently told by her physician that she had diabetes and would likely be diabetic for the rest of her life. When she heard her doctor's diagnosis, she was shocked.

Something must have happened in the past 30 years because when she was 20, she could eat anything, exercise if she wanted, and was always thin and healthy. After hearing both of these stories, I introduced the young man to the woman and let them visit for a few minutes. The need to adopt a healthy lifestyle is important for all ages.

You can do this; others already have. The long life spans of Mormons and Seventh-Day Adventists show that it is possible. Studies of diabetics, cardiac patients, cancer patients, obese people, children, college students, adults, and even seniors have shown that regular exercise and a healthy diet can be achieved at any age and in any health condition. More importantly, these new behaviors can be maintained for years.

In the 1900s the advent of antibiotics dramatically changed public health and death as it was then known. Infectious diseases, which used to be responsible for almost 30% of all deaths at that time, are now responsible for just 2% of deaths.[33] This dramatic improvement in public health can be repeated. The adoption of a healthy lifestyle can have a greater national impact on chronic disease and death than any other single factor known in all of medicine. If Americans will adopt healthy lifestyles, there will be a public health revolution.

POINTS TO REMEMBER

- An unhealthy lifestyle is the main cause of most cases of chronic diseases.

- A healthy lifestyle will most likely extend the length of your life.

- A healthy lifestyle can reduce the degree of poor health most people have at the end of life. It can help you live a high-quality, active life to the very end.

- It isn't easy, but you can change your lifestyle; others already have.

Let Science Be Your Guide

There are in fact two things, science and opinion;
the former begets knowledge, the latter ignorance.
—Hippocrates

IMAGINE YOU RECEIVE A JIGSAW PUZZLE AS A GIFT. This is no ordinary puzzle! It requires 50,000 individual pieces, but most of them are missing, and some of the pieces you do have are blank. But you have a picture of what the final puzzle is supposed to look like, so you begin working on the puzzle. You find a few pieces that fit, but progress is painfully slow—sometimes the pieces appear to fit one way, but later you find they were upside down or located in the wrong spot. Still, you know that if you work long enough and get enough pieces, you will begin to see a very rough image of the final picture.

Researchers trying to understand what is needed for good health are working to solve a similar puzzle. They know what the final picture is: a long and high-quality life free from debilitating chronic diseases. But the process of putting the puzzle together is difficult. As you will learn in this chapter, the process of finding the puzzle pieces and making them fit together is expensive, painfully slow, and complicated by apparently contradictory research. Often the research is misinterpreted by the media, and ongoing research is continually being added to what is already known.

Finding Puzzle Pieces

One of the best ways to complete a puzzle is to look closely at the final picture and try to determine which pieces fit where. For scientists this means finding groups of people who live long, high-quality lives and then studying them. Every year in the United States, 37% of all deaths result from cardiovascular diseases, such as heart attacks and strokes, and another 23% of all deaths are caused by cancer.[1] On average in the United States, males live to the age of 74 and females to the age of 80. How do these numbers compare to other countries? Are there other places on earth where people live longer and have fewer chronic diseases? These are the questions researchers have been asking for years.

The search for answers to these questions has led to the discovery of many of the puzzle pieces. For example, a study of men from the United States, Finland, the Netherlands, Italy, the former Yugoslavia, Greece, and Japan showed very large differences in the number of heart disease deaths. Men in Finland were 6.5 times more likely to die of heart disease than men in Japan.[2] Other studies have looked at differences in the occurrence of cancer and cancer deaths, obesity, diabetes, Alzheimer's, and many other conditions.[3]

Once a specific group of people is identified as being at either high or low risk for any condition, the search for puzzle pieces intensifies. For example, if scientists find that Japanese men have much lower rates of heart disease than American men do, the scientists then attempt to discover why Japanese men have a lower risk for heart disease. In order to do this, the scientists might look at differences in diet, exercise, genetics, or environment. Researchers have developed different research tools to identify these pieces and determine how they fit together.

The Tools

Fifty years ago, 5,209 healthy, middle-aged residents of Framingham, Massachusetts, were selected to be part of a study to help determine why so many people in the country were dying from heart disease. At the beginning of the study, these residents volunteered to have extensive physical exams and lab tests. This baseline medical information was stored, and every few years the researchers would return and gather more medical information from these same residents.

After 20 years, many of the original subjects in the study had passed away. For each of the deceased, an exact cause of death was determined. When the researchers looked at the early medical records for all the study participants who had died from heart disease, for example, they were amazed to find that the deceased were much more likely to be from among those whose early records included a diagnosis of high blood pressure or high blood cholesterol. When those who smoked or were overweight were excluded from the data, high blood pressure and high blood cholesterol were still very good indicators for cause of death.

This famous study is called the Framingham Heart Study[4] and is an example of a *cohort study*—a study that follows a large group of people over a long period of time until some of the participants develop specific diseases or die from certain causes. The information and research findings from the Framingham Heart Study have been published in over 1,000 scientific articles and have forever changed what we know about the prevention of heart disease and cancer.

Though the study was started over 50 years ago and the original researchers have died, data from the Framingham Heart Study is still providing valuable information because medical data has since been gathered from the children, grandchildren, and even great-grandchildren of the original study participants. All this information has been combined with results from other cohort studies to produce a large number of puzzle pieces.

The Framingham study was completed at a time when very little was known about the importance of a healthy diet and physical activity. Since the study was begun, other cohort studies have been used to investigate all sorts of diseases in a wide variety of populations. Right now there are hundreds of cohort studies being conducted in countries around the world. Each of these studies follows the same format—researchers gather health data from people, they wait to see what happens to the participants, and then they use the data to identify trends in or relationships among health risk factors. These studies are extremely hard to conduct and can cost millions of dollars; some studies have over 300,000 participants who are measured and tracked for decades. Perhaps you are wondering who pays for all of these expensive studies. You do! Virtually all large cohort studies are funded with federal and state tax dollars. However, as you will learn in this book, this investment has been a very good use of taxpayer dollars.

A *case-control study* is another common research tool that works like a cohort study but in reverse. Individuals with certain diseases are paired with similar individuals who don't have the disease. For example, if a researcher wanted to know why so many Americans are obese, that researcher would locate several hundred obese individuals; locate several hundred volunteers of similar age, gender, or race who are not obese; and then the researcher would ask both groups about their nutrition and exercise habits, family medical history, or anything else that might cause obesity. Lastly, the researcher would compare calories consumed or exercise habits between the two groups to see if there is any difference.

Unfortunately, if a cohort or case-control study suggests that lack of exercise is related to obesity, this does not provide absolute proof. It is difficult to determine which comes first: Do obese individuals become obese because they were first sedentary or do individuals become obese for other reasons and then become sedentary? Unless researchers conduct a randomized clinical trial, it is very difficult to know.

In a *randomized clinical trial*, volunteers are randomly assigned to either a control group or a group that gets some sort of intervention or drug. For example, a randomized clinical trial could be conducted to see what happens to people when they become really lazy. A group of volunteers could be assigned to be in a treatment group that gets to sit around all day and be lazy or a control group whose members continue to live their normal lives. Members of both groups would have to eat exactly the same amounts of food. After several months, the researcher would see if there are any differences between the two groups. More than likely, the sedentary group of participants will have gained more weight than the control group, and the researcher could state that being sedentary most likely leads to weight gain. After all, the only difference between the two groups is that one became sedentary. Randomized clinical trials are one of the more powerful tools used to determine the keys to good health. Unfortunately, much of what we do to maintain good health does not come from good science; it comes from tradition, religious beliefs, cultural pressure, or personal experience.

• •

INSIDE THE ALDANA HOME ▶▶▶ *When I was growing up, I used to have a few warts on the back of my hand. One day I ate a whole bag of black licorice and within a week or two, I noticed that the warts disappeared, and I haven't seen them since. From that experience, I have developed several possible explanations to explain why the warts went away: something in the licorice made them go away, something caused my immune system to suddenly get the upper hand on wart-causing viruses, or somehow the warts spontaneously disappeared at about the same time I ate the licorice (and likely would have disappeared regardless of what I had eaten).*

So which one is correct? I have no idea, but in my opinion, I think it was simply spontaneous remission. The warts would have gone away regardless of what I had eaten. My experience and knowledge about warts and licorice makes me believe this way, but without scientific evidence, I could easily be wrong. In the absence of any good scientific information, the only thing left is opinion, and even though personal opinions are the most unreliable source of health information, it is the source of much of the advice we hear from friends, neighbors, and the media.

. . . .

Even the Researchers Seem Confused

Cohort and case-control studies and randomized clinical trials are used regularly to try to locate pieces of the healthy lifestyle puzzle. But even with these tools, it isn't easy to solve the puzzle. Have you ever heard a news report that says some food or lifestyle is really good for you only to find out months or years later that the earlier information was not correct? Why does this happen? Why can't scientists agree with each other and give us accurate pieces of the puzzle, or at least keep quiet until they have it all figured out? For those who are trying to live a healthy lifestyle, this contradictory information is a major source of frustration.

There are several very good reasons why things seem so confusing. Since no one has all the pieces, what researchers think might be correct can end up being wrong. And even though researchers have great tools and can do clever, creative studies, sometimes the results from different studies on the same topic don't agree.

For example, there are a large number of both cohort and case-control studies that have evaluated the relationship between exercise and breast cancer. Many researchers have compared the number of breast cancer cases between people who do exercise and people who do not exercise. Figure 2.1 shows the results from 34 different studies that compared the rates of breast cancer between women who exercised regularly, with breast cancer rates among women who didn't.[5]

The first study listed in the figure was completed in Finland. The little dot out to the far right of the word *Finland* is placed in the higher risk area, suggesting that women in this study who exercised had a higher risk of getting breast cancer than women who did not. That's right, you read correctly—the first few studies in the figure report a higher risk of beast cancer for women who exercised. All told, there are six studies that reported a slightly higher risk of breast cancer for women who exercised regularly. These six studies are represented by the six dots in the higher risk side of the figure.

Study	Lower Risk							Same Risk		Higher Risk
	.3	.4	.5	.6	.7	.8	.9	1	1.5	2
Cohort Studies										
Finland									•	
Massachusetts, U.S.										•
United States								•		
Seventh-Day Adventists, U.S.				•						
Pennsylvania, U.S.				•						
U.S. Nurses								•		
U.S. Nurses								•		
U.S. Nurses					•					
Iowa, U.S.						•				
United States, Former College Athletes			•							
Shanghai, China					•					
United States, Former College Athletes				•						
Case-Control Studies										
United States, Age 40 and Under			•							
Alberta, Canada					•					
United States: ME, MA, NH, WI			•							
Washington, U.S.				•						
United States: Occupations 4 states							•			
Washington, U.S.						•				
United States, Occupations									•	
Atlanta, GA; Central NJ; Seattle, WA; U.S.								•		
United States, Activity at Age 12						•				
Los Angeles County, CA, U.S.			•							
Cape Cod, MA, U.S.						•				
Sweden						•				
WI, MA, ME, NH, U.S.			•							
Amsterdam, The Netherlands					•					
Istanbul, Turkey							•			
New York, U.S.								•		
Nagoya, Japan					•					
Milan, Italy					•					
Gifu, Japan			•							
Miian, Italy				•						
Tsukubu, Japan	•									
Switzerland	•									

Figure 2.1 Results of studies that looked at the risk of breast cancer for those who are physically active

Two studies showed that there was no difference in breast cancer risk between exercisers and non-exercisers (dots on the center line), while the rest of the studies in the figure (26 of them) showed that exercisers have a lower risk of breast cancer. On average, this last group of studies showed that exercisers have about half the risk of getting breast cancer than non-exercisers. So what are you to believe? A few studies demonstrated that exercisers have more risk, a few showed the risk is the same, and the vast majority of studies showed that exercisers have about half the risk.

With this information, you now know almost all there is to know about the relationship between exercise and beast cancer. If someone were to ask you if you think exercise helps prevent breast cancer, how would you respond? The best answer might be something like, "Exercise *most likely* lowers a person's risk of getting breast cancer." Now you are starting to sound like a scientist. This example of contradictory research is not unique. Research on several health issues has produced findings that are both favorable and unfavorable.

Conflicting scientific findings are only partially to blame for the confusion felt by the public. When scientists want to report important findings, they write an article about a study they have done. This report is carefully reviewed by several experts, and if the experts approve of the study methods, they recommend that the report be published in a scientific journal. The only way the typical American will ever hear about the study is if he or she reads the scientific journal or if someone in the media reads the journal and decides to do a story about it. This is where it can get confusing.

Journalists are paid to write stories that people will pay to read or watch on television. Therefore, journalists need to write stories that are of interest to readers and viewers, so sometimes they have to jazz up the studies to make them a little more interesting. Look back at Figure 2.1 (the summary of all the studies on exercise and breast cancer). If you were a journalist needing to write stories that sell and the research from Finland was just published, you could write an article entitled, "Study shows exercise can cause breast cancer." The title is accurate and, more than likely, will draw many people to the story. The title alone does no harm—so long as the article presents the results of the study in context with the rest of what is known about exercise and breast cancer, something a good journalist would do. But many times this does not happen, and if it does happen but the public doesn't read the article, the title of the article might be all the public remembers about the study. It would be far more accurate—and clearly more boring—to entitle the article, "Exercise and breast cancer study at odds with most other studies."

By far the most confusing and outright deceptive health information comes from advertising and marketing campaigns from the food, supplement, tobacco, alcohol, and exercise industries. Take the dairy industry, for example. Milk consumption is a classic example of the confusion we've been talking about because the scientific research both supports and discourages milk consumption. We've all heard that "milk does a body good" because we've heard the advertisements and seen the marketing efforts. We also know that famous people drink whole milk because we see them on billboards and in ads with milk mustaches on their upper lips. And while the dairy industry is quick to report the research that shows the benefits of milk consumption, like reduced risk of osteoporosis,[6] have you heard anything about the numerous and convincing research studies that link whole-milk consumption with prostate and ovarian cancer?

The dairy industry is passionate about selling milk and milk products. They also fund a considerable amount of milk-related research. The fact that some have suggested that researchers who are paid by the milk industry to conduct research on milk are under pressure to report only favorable findings that connect milk consumption with good health[7] only adds to the confusion about what information we can trust. A scientific summary of what we know about milk will be provided later in this book; for now, you should know that most of the puzzle pieces related to the benefits of milk for adults are still undiscovered or not fully understood.

Despite the scientific evidence that supports the need to consume whole grains and cereals, food makers claim that Chocolate Frosted Sugar Bombs breakfast cereal is part of a healthy breakfast.

One of the unfortunate side effects of being a citizen in a capitalistic society such as the United States is that aggressive producers of goods have the financial need to convince citizens to purchase their products. If you haven't watched morning cartoons in a while, you haven't missed much; the cartoons and food commercials are about the same. Despite the scientific evidence that supports the need to consume whole grains and cereals, food makers claim that Chocolate Frosted Sugar Bombs breakfast cereal is part of a healthy breakfast. This might be true if a small bowl of the cereal were consumed with some whole wheat toast and fruit, but most children, including mine, will fill up on several bowls of the cereal and never get to the toast and fruit—they'd do the same for lunch and dinner if they were permitted to.

This forceful marketing only adds to the confusion we feel about the guidelines for good health. As a general rule of thumb, you are likely better off if you make health decisions based on information from legitimate public organizations such as governments, nonprofit organizations, and colleges or universities. These groups may be the most reliable sources of health information because they're usually not supported by for-profit companies, such as drug or insurance companies, who are trying to sell you something.

"Choose Ye This Day"

Marketing campaigns, media reports and articles, comments by scientists, and outright deception can influence what we eat. In addition to these factors, many faith-based communities have specific dietary guidelines that are part of their religious observance. All these religiously based dietary codes of conduct predate any scientific evidence about healthy diets. Seventh-Day Adventists and some Buddhist groups are encouraged to be vegetarians; Mormons have a doctrine that recommends a diet based on whole grains, fruits and vegetables, and little meat. Most conservative and orthodox Jews follow the biblical teachings to avoid meat from unclean animals like pork and to have their meat butchered by a trained observant or licensed Jewish slaughterer.

So how does one reconcile religious dietary doctrines with modern science? Luckily, you don't have to; a close look at the scientific literature shows that science supports most religious doctrines of vegetarian living, low consumption of meat, and lots of whole grains, fruits, and vegetables. In other words, it appears that these religious doctrines have been accurate all along.

With large numbers of active members, these various religious groups provide researchers with unique opportunities to study the impact of healthy diets on death and disease. Research on Seventh-Day Adventists and Mormons shows that members of these religions live considerably longer than average and have much lower rates of many chronic diseases.[8-9] So far, the dietary doctrines of many common faith communities match up very well with what we now know are good health practices. However, if some religious group decided that its members should eat only highly processed foods like cheese puffs, chocolate, ice cream, and cake, there would be a conflict between religious beliefs and science, although I know many children and adults who would want to convert.

Future Fine Tuning

When it comes to the importance of a healthy lifestyle in the prevention of chronic diseases and the attainment of a high-quality life, enough puzzle pieces have been found to give us a fairly good picture of what our diets and exercise patterns should be. After all, we know what the final picture is; we just need to identify the steps required to get there. The Healthy Eating Pyramid and exercise recommendations found in chapter 1 of this book are based on enormous amounts of scientific research, with no influence from groups wanting to profit from the recommendations.

But even though this research is mostly free from financial conflicts of interest, the recommendations summarized in this book will undergo change in the future. As more and more puzzle pieces are found and connected with other known scientific findings, our understanding of the body's nutritional requirements will undergo small but continual changes, a constant process of fine tuning.

Exercise is always going to be required for good health, and at present, the best recommendation is to accumulate 30 minutes of moderate-intensity activity on most, preferably all, days of the week. The best recommendations for diet include the following:

- Eat a minimum of five servings of fruits and/or vegetables every day.
- Eat whole grain breads, cereals, and other high-fiber foods.
- Limit the consumption of red meat to no more than once a week (fish, poultry, and eggs are excellent alternatives).
- Consume nuts and beans regularly.
- Limit consumption of saturated fat.
- Avoid all trans fats.

This description of a healthy diet might appear to be fairly complicated, but it is not. In general, you should eat whole foods that are close to their natural form. And even though these recommendations will undergo some changes, they represent a fairly complete picture of the diet puzzle—much of the fine tuning in the future will likely demonstrate that the benefits of a healthy diet are more dramatic than previously thought.

For some people, these current recommendations read like morphine in print, causing an almost immediate sensation of sleepiness and overall apathy. That's not surprising. The recommendations are simply general conclusions in the form of one-line summaries of all that is known about healthy living, written by scientists and researchers who have devoted their entire professional lives to understanding how to help the body stay healthy; these summaries do not reveal the good stuff—the irrefutable evidence supporting the relationship between diet, exercise, and good health or all the things that can be done to change lifestyles.

Friends and relatives who see me exercising with my family or eating a healthy meal often ask me how I can stay motivated to live a healthy lifestyle. I honestly feel that if they knew what I know about lifestyle and good health, they would probably do the same; to do otherwise would go contrary to just about all the scientific evidence we have today. By reading the rest of this book, you will know what I and other researchers know; you will see that the good stuff behind the recommendations gives you a perspective that will forever change what you think about your health. The real challenge is doing something about it because, despite all the amazing scientific findings, many people suffer from "I-don't-care-itis," a common condition that we'll discuss more in chapter 3.

POINTS TO REMEMBER

- Trying to figure out what is necessary for good health is a complex puzzle.

- Even though scientists use the best tools available, discovering the truth about good health is not easy; there are often contradictory findings.

- The media and aggressive marketing tactics make it difficult for the public to separate fact from fiction.

- The current recommendations for regular physical activity and good nutrition will continue to undergo refinements.

3

I-Don't-Care-itis: The Most Common Health Problem in America

Some day healthy people are going to feel really
stupid, lying in hospital beds dying of nothing.
—Author Unknown

IF YOU ARE A TYPICAL YOUNG OR MIDDLE-AGED ADULT, you are not likely to be suffering from pain or symptoms of chronic disease of any sort. You feel healthy, your physician gives you a clean bill of health, and you feel like you can eat whatever you want, exercise or not, and you feel fine either way. Why should you be concerned about your health if you feel fine?

And since the really big, lifesaving benefits associated with a healthy lifestyle are waiting for you in the future, why should you be concerned about your future health now? Sure, there are some great immediate benefits of a healthy lifestyle, like weight loss, improved fitness, increased energy, and improved sleep quality, but you won't experience the big benefits for many years. So why worry about something that won't happen for a long time? This is a great question and the leading cause of I-don't-care-itis.

I-don't-care-itis is a common condition in which an individual has no interest in adopting a healthy lifestyle. There are many common symptoms of I-don't-care-itis. These symptoms tend to go away as you get older, they are almost always unrecognized by those who have them, and they generally clear up quickly once dietary and exercise habits are improved. Ask yourself the following questions:

- Do you believe that the food and lifestyle traditions of your family and culture are okay because that's the way it's always been?

- Do you feel threatened when someone suggests that you could be healthier if you changed the way you eat?

- Do you feel discouraged because you tried to make changes before, but you failed?

- Do you think that you already have a healthy lifestyle and don't need to change anything?

- Do you feel it is worth it to maintain your current food and exercise habits even though they may shorten your life by more than ten years?

- Do you believe that there is nothing wrong with your current lifestyle so "why fix it if it ain't broke"?

If you answered yes to any of these questions, you may have I-don't-care-itis. You are not alone; in fact, you are in the majority. Most Americans (83%) don't have a healthy diet, and many Americans (67%) don't get enough exercise to enjoy the benefits. If you fall into this category, the pages you are about to read will hopefully help convince you to think seriously about the future and make meaningful lifestyle changes.

The Youthful Attitude of Immortality

It is in human nature to push the envelope—to keep doing something a little faster or a little more dangerous until something happens. Many older adults have already discovered their limits and no longer have the need to push their boundaries. For example, most adults don't like staying up all night. They've learned that the zombie-like feeling they have the next day is worse than the enjoyment they get out of staying up.

Many of us have played aggressively with an open fire or heat source until we were burned; then we backed off a bit. Many of us have gotten increasingly reckless when riding a bicycle or driving a car until something bad happened. At that instant we discovered our limits. Pain definitely lets us know where our limits are. Each of us has to readjust our sense of immortality to better reflect our mortal nature. In other words, if we don't learn quickly where the limits are, we will suffer the consequences, be seriously injured, or even suffer premature death, the ultimate experience of mortality.

There is one small problem, however. When playing with fire, the limits of what we can and cannot do are quickly and painfully discovered; the pain associated with eating an extremely unhealthy diet is most often not experienced during the act. To the contrary, we very much enjoy unhealthy foods because they taste so good.

Preventing common chronic diseases and premature death later in life requires that you take action now, even though you have no symptoms of chronic diseases.

Most likely, any life-threatening pain won't be felt for many, many years, so we have a tendency not to worry about the future, just as in the story of the grasshopper and the ant. The ant works hard in the withering heat all summer long, building his house and laying up supplies for the winter. The grasshopper thinks he's a fool and laughs and dances and plays the summer away. Come winter, the ant is warm and well fed, but the grasshopper has no food or shelter, so he dies out in the cold. The ant prevented hunger and cold by preparing early, even though he was neither hungry nor cold at the time. Preventing common chronic diseases and premature death later in life requires that you take action now, even though you have no symptoms of chronic diseases.

Let's use the following ancestor worksheet in Figure 3.1 to help personalize the need to start making changes now. The worksheet shows you, your parents, your grandparents, and your great-grandparents. For your relatives who have passed away, write down the causes of their deaths on the lines above their names. If you don't know, now would be a great time to ask.

Based on U.S. death data, we know that of the 2.5 million people who died in 2002, 37% died from complications of cardiovascular diseases, 23% died of cancer, and 3% died of diabetes.[1] Your worksheet may show that none of the deaths in your immediate family were caused by any of these diseases, but, on average, individual pedigrees will mirror national trends,

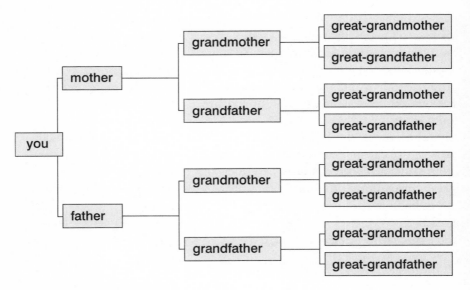

Figure 3.1 Ancestor worksheet

and most individuals are likely to have a pedigree that includes relatives who died prematurely or suffered from largely preventable diseases.

Most cases of chronic disease are caused by lifestyle factors. This also means that most deaths due to chronic diseases are lifestyle related. There is no way to know for sure if the deaths in your family were due to an unhealthy lifestyle, but, on average, most deaths are the result of lifestyle choices—especially for those who live and die in the United States.

This exercise helps link the importance of healthy living to you and your family members. It helps you realize that the way you live your life now will directly impact your future, for better or for worse. Most often our learned behaviors and environment have a greater impact on our health than genetics do.

Welcome to America

In 1951, the Pentagon dispatched physicians to Korea with the grisly task of studying the fatal wounds of soldiers who had died in combat during the Korean War. Over 2,000 autopsies were performed on soldiers who had been athletic and apparently looked healthy before death. The doctors began seeing signs of coronary heart disease among the soldiers.[2] This was completely unexpected, since heart disease at that time was known as a disease that affected the elderly, not 22-year-old men. The pathologists decided to keep track of the number of soldiers that had evidence of heart disease.

Healthy arteries have an inner surface that is thin and very smooth, and the artery is open. Smooth surfaces are required if blood is to flow unimpeded to the various cells of the body. If the inner surface of an artery is not smooth, the blood can deposit a plaque-like substance on the surface. Surrounding this inner, smooth layer of an artery is a layer of smooth muscle that can contract and expand as blood pressure and the demands of the body change. Instead of finding smooth surfaces within the arteries of the hearts of the soldiers, researchers found fibrous, fatty yellow streaks or deposits. The muscle layer of the arteries had grown abnormally, extending into the artery. In many of the casualties, the fatty streaks had already grown into lesions (abnormal growths that contain deposits of fats and cholesterol referred to as plaque). Once established, lesions continue to grow and develop, causing the opening inside the artery to get smaller and smaller. This is called atherosclerosis, and it leads to heart disease.

Amazingly, 77% of the American Korean War casualties examined showed dramatic evidence of coronary heart disease. The researchers were stunned by this finding. How could young, apparently healthy men have advanced stages of heart disease? The medical community was shocked because it appeared that heart disease was an outcome of a process that may have started in childhood.

Even though the overall rates of heart disease in the United States have declined since the Korean War, recent studies of young adults suggest that the disease process is still well underway in most young adults. In 1993, an autopsy study of young U.S. men who had died in accidents was conducted. It found that out of 111 young males, 78% were found to have heart disease rates identical to those found among the Korean War casualties.[3]

Among the young men who had evidence of disease, 30% had vessels that were more than half closed. Similar findings have been seen in young women, and it is not just vessels of the heart that are affected. Using special equipment, physicians documented that fatty streaks and lesions were also found in neck arteries of living young adults and even teenagers.[4-6] These particular deposits pose no immediate threat, but they likely will continue to progress, and as the flow of blood becomes increasingly blocked, a heart attack, stroke, or other vessel-related problem will eventually result.

Cardiovascular disease starts early in life, progressively worsens, and is responsible for more deaths than any other disease. But this is not the case for everyone. Before 1970, autopsies conducted on deceased Japanese citizens rarely showed any signs of artery disease, fatty streaks, or lesions. As Japan has begun adopting American foods and lifestyles (becoming Westernized), the average amount of blood cholesterol and body fat in the typical Japanese citizen has increased significantly. From 1952 to 1994, Japanese children increased their dietary fat from 13% to 33%, almost a 300% increase.[7] During this same time, the number of cases of cardiovascular diseases in Japanese adults increased 400%.[8]

Studies of native Japanese and Japanese-Americans show that the high rates of cardiovascular disease in the United States are directly related to our American lifestyle. By following rates of heart disease among Japanese citizens who live in Japan, citizens who have migrated to Hawaii, and citizens who have migrated to California, the connection between the most common killer and the American lifestyle becomes very clear. Native Japanese had almost no cases of heart disease, disease rates among Japanese men in Hawaii were dramatically greater than those in Japan, and those who had migrated to California had 50% more heart disease than those in Hawaii.[9] The cause of this disease is obviously related to the degree to which the immigrants adopted the lifestyle of their new country. These results cannot be caused by genetics because the changes in heart disease rates occurred within one generation.

You feel fine, you are having a normal day, suddenly you feel severe chest and neck pain, and you die—that quickly.

It's not just Japanese Americans who develop these diseases. Some of the healthiest people on earth eat a Mediterranean-type diet that is high in fruits, vegetables, and healthy oils and low in saturated fat. Portuguese adults and children are slowly abandoning their traditional Mediterranean diet and are adopting Western diets by eating more saturated fat, which causes them to have higher blood cholesterol and, eventually, cardiovascular disease.[10]

Similar changes occur in immigrants who come to the United States. African-Americans, Mexican-Americans, Latin Americans, Pacific Islanders, and many other ethnic groups who migrate to America and replace their native foods and lifestyles with American foods and lifestyles initiate the cardiovascular disease process. If these newest members of American society would bring their native food traditions with them and not change them, they would not experience the chronic diseases and premature death experienced by most Americans. Unfortunately, in the process of becoming American citizens, many migrants adopt American ways, learn to live like Americans, and, with time, die like Americans.

Chronic Diseases, Silent and Unseen

Whenever the news media reports on a passenger jet that has experienced difficulties and crashed, it is almost always front-page news in papers across America. What would the reaction be if seven fully loaded 747s crashed in a single day, killing all on board? What if this terrible tragedy were repeated every single day for an entire year? The total of all these fatalities is still slightly less than the total number of deaths in the United States that are caused by cardiovascular disease each year.

Cardiovascular disease is the number one cause of death. It includes any disease that is brought on by blocked, weakened, or hardened arteries; these primarily include heart disease and stroke. A common misconception is that it is a man's disease; however, women are more likely to die of a heart attack or a stroke than men are.

Even though cardiovascular disease is common and its main causes are known, it is still hard to live a healthy lifestyle in order to prevent it. This is partially because cardiovascular disease is very sneaky; it gives no warning or notice that it is developing. There is no pain, and there are no signs or symptoms of the disease, even though the disease may be well underway. Not until the disease is so severe that blood flow has been dramatically reduced do you begin to notice anything is wrong.

In half of the cardiovascular disease deaths that occur each year, the first signs that anything is wrong are sudden cardiac arrest and death.[11] You feel fine, you are having a normal day, suddenly you feel severe chest and neck pain, and you die—that quickly. In these cases, you get no second chances, no time to vow to change your ways, no opportunity to recommit to your exercise program, no last hugs and kisses for the ones you love; it's painful, it's quick, and it's often preventable.

In the early days of the automobile, windshields were made out of regular plate glass and there were no seat belts. Hundreds of thousands of people worldwide died from relatively minor accidents when they were mortally injured from the broken glass. At the time, this was thought to be an act of God. After all, it was viewed as an unavoidable accident. Today, safety glass, seat belts, and air bags have eliminated almost all deaths from minor automobile collisions because these deaths are preventable, not acts of God.

So, does this mean that sudden death due to cardiovascular disease is an act of God? Not likely. Those with healthy body weight and a good diet who avoid tobacco use and exercise regularly can prevent most cases of cardiovascular disease from developing, stop it if it has already begun, and even reverse blockage that may have already occurred.[12-14]

If you take the U.S. population and evaluate their arteries based on age, you get the image shown in Figure 3.2. The circle above each age group shows the level of artery blockage that is typical for Americans in that age group.

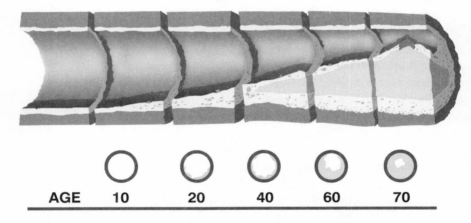

| AGE | 10 | 20 | 40 | 60 | 70 |

Figure 3.2 Age and degree of atherosclerosis in the United States

There are exceptions to this graph, but, in general, it represents the U.S. population. If you locate your age group in the figure, you can see the level of artery disease that is most common among people your age. It appears that as you get older, your arteries get more and more blocked, but it is not age that causes the blockage; it is exposure to a Western lifestyle.

If this same figure were drawn using rural native Asians or Europeans who still consume a Mediterranean-type diet, the clean arteries at the age of 10 would also be typical of arteries in later decades of life. Every year of eating a Western diet and avoiding physical activity adds to the total amount of vessel disease a person develops.

What about Children?

Since the Korean autopsy study, researchers have been wondering when and how cardiovascular disease gets started. If 20-year-old soldiers have advanced levels of the disease, it must start sometime before then.

To explore this question, the U.S. government spent millions of federal tax dollars to finance the longest and most detailed study of children in the world.[15–16]

In 1972, all the black and white children of the town of Bogalusa, Louisiana, were invited to participate in a large cohort study. The purpose of the study was to understand the early natural history of coronary artery disease. Researchers gathered medical and health information from the children, treated those who needed any medial treatment, and then let the children live their lives.

After 30 to 40 years, most of these children had grown up, started families, gotten jobs, and experienced periodic health issues. As they aged, more and more acquired various chronic diseases. Researchers then went back to the childhood data to determine which factors might predict who would have medical problems later in life. This research has resulted in more than 700 publications and three textbooks on child health, and researchers continue to follow 14,000 children and young adults. You can probably guess what they have found.

- Heart disease starts in children and is evident at 5 to 8 years of age.
- Poor diet and lack of physical activity lead to high blood cholesterol, high blood pressure, and obesity, which likely cause heart disease to start in children.
- Unhealthy lifestyles and behaviors that influence cardiovascular disease are learned and begin early in life.
- If chronic diseases are to be prevented in adults, healthy lifestyles should be adopted in childhood.

It is depressing to think that what we feed our children has a very good chance of causing their premature death later in life. But there is some good news—at least your hard-earned federal tax dollars have been put to very good use. Researchers from around the world and around the United States have completed similar studies on children and have all come to similar conclusions: cardiovascular disease starts early in life and advances quickly when a person is overweight or obese or has elevated cholesterol.[17–23]

There is even some evidence of the disease when we go back to the very beginning of human development, when the fetus is developing; the major arteries of some miscarried fetuses showed fatty streaks, the beginning stage of artery disease.[24] This is due to the genetic makeup and nutritional status of the mother. You've heard the saying that you are what you eat; well, the corollary to this is that your children are what you eat, and your unborn child is what you eat.

We know a lot about good health and disease prevention, but the difficult part of knowing all this information is convincing ourselves of the need to change. The information gleaned from these studies could prevent hundreds of thousands of premature deaths from cardiovascular disease and stroke if people would just modify their eating and physical activity habits. In fact, despite all the fantastic medical advancements, the greatest improvements in public health will come from lifestyle change, not from more advanced treatments or medications.

War Games

A healthy lifestyle doesn't prevent just cardiovascular disease. Cancer, the number two killer in America, is the next most common chronic disease that is lifestyle related, mostly preventable, and strongly related to diet, physical activity, and tobacco use. Presently, one out of every three American adults will get cancer, and 23% of all Americans will die of it. Most oncologists (cancer doctors) know that the longer you live, the more likely you are to get cancer because the diseases that are classified as cancers are all opportunists.

Cancer is any malignant growth or tumor caused by abnormal and uncontrolled cell division. The abnormal cell division is caused by abnormal cell DNA. DNA can be damaged in one of two ways: a spontaneous error can get started during normal cell division, or free radicals produced by our own bodies or in the foods we consume can damage DNA. The whole cancer process is just one great big, ongoing battle; the battle starts when we are just fetuses developing in our mothers' wombs and continues until we die. It goes on every day and night for our entire lives.

Right now, while you are reading these words, the battle is raging. It's us against abnormal DNA. The chapter on fruits, vegetables, and whole grains will talk more about the details of this battle and what you can do to increase your chances of winning, but for now it is important to know who the players are.

The bad guys are free radicals. These are not fringe political groups who may advocate using extreme measures to incite political unrest—they are tiny little molecules that are unhappy because they are missing an electron, and they won't be happy until they get one. They will use any means possible to satisfy their need for an electron; they may steal, borrow, or even kill for one.

Defending us in this battle against abnormal DNA is an array of specialized warriors, each possessing a select set of skills and equipment. These warriors can stop the cancer process at its inception, during its growth, and even when it might be spreading. Most of these good guys are designed to stop cancer very early in the process, even before any DNA is attacked. Once an abnormal DNA has multiplied and begun to spread, the war is not lost, but the battle has reached a climax. If the battle reaches this point, and it does in one out of every three adults who are afflicted with cancer, the conflict escalates to nuclear warfare when medical professionals bring out the weapons of mass destruction: radiation therapy, chemotherapy, and surgery.

Just like cardiovascular disease, cancer can take a lifetime to develop. Once a cancer begins to spread, it grows quickly, and medical care is the only viable treatment option. If you are suffering from I-don't-care-itis, you may feel little sense of urgency or concern about cancer because it affects mostly older adults, takes a lifetime of defending against abnormal DNA, and becomes a problem only if your body fails to keep abnormal DNA under control.

People who will increase their fruit and vegetable consumption from two servings a day to five servings a day can cut the risk of getting many cancers by half.

Any field commander who enters battle with an insufficient number of troops, inferior equipment, an inadequate fuel supply, or a limited number of ways to attack the enemy would certainly be much more vulnerable to defeat. This is precisely what happens when you eat a typical American diet consisting of foods high in fat, refined flour, and sugar and low in fruits, vegetables, and whole grains. Only 22% of Americans consume five servings of fruits and vegetables per day.[25]

The cancer prevention battle raging in the bodies of most Americans is poorly equipped and manned, which is one reason cancer is the second leading cause of death in the United States. This does not have to be the case. Long-term epidemiological data shows that people who will increase their fruit and vegetable consumption from two servings a day to five servings a day can cut the risk of getting many types of cancer by half.[26] This is clear evidence that a good diet can tip the odds of a military conquest in your favor.

Smokers are at a definite military disadvantage. One of the largest sources of free radicals is tobacco smoke. It is not uncommon for a person to smoke two to three packs of cigarettes a day and have a diet that includes almost no fruits and vegetables or whole grains. In this case, the tobacco smoke dramatically increases the number of free radicals, and the poor diet reduces a person's ability to defend against cancer. This double whammy is like going to war with too few troops and no supplies. It is easy to see what the outcome of the battle will be.

On average, cigarette smokers die 14 years earlier than nonsmokers.[27] It is extremely difficult for many smokers to quit, but that doesn't mean that smokers can't eat well. Smokers should be assisted in every possible way to quit, but if they do not, they can still reduce some of their cancer risk by eating a healthy diet and exercising.

Fix Me Up, Doc

Let's suppose you really don't care about your diet or your physical activity level because you have seen the miraculous medical procedures that can be performed on people with chronic diseases, especially cardiovascular disease. After all, bypass surgery, angioplasty (balloons and stents inserted in the blocked artery), and medications have been used for years and have improved life for many of those with cardiovascular disease. This "fix me up, Doc" attitude is very common; eat whatever you want, exercise only if you really want to, and, if you do have heart problems, just have the doctor fix you up. This is surely an easy approach to perceived high-quality living, but in all fairness, an objective view of the facts goes a long way toward changing this attitude.

The effectiveness of medical care in the United States is better than anywhere else in the world.[28] If you need medical care, this is the place; if you need treatment for cardiovascular disease, you are in luck because your options are plentiful. This is good news if you are among the half of all people with heart disease who survive the initial attack. If you are in the other half, well, you won't need any of these fantastic medical procedures.

Medications have always been used to treat cardiovascular disease, but the best results come from the creative techniques doctors have devised to fix the problem. Surgeons figured out how to take a vein out of one part of a person's body and use it to reroute blood around a blocked part of an artery to the heart. These bypasses require open-heart surgery, and more than half a million people in the United States have this procedure each year.

Rather than bypass plugged arteries, physicians can also insert a tiny plastic tube (catheter) into your arteries, slide it into your heart to the place where the blockage is located, and inflate a little balloon to push the blockage out of the way. This procedure is called an angioplasty. Besides balloons, there are also tiny spinning razor blades that can slice up the blockage (the roto-rooter method), and lasers that can vaporize the blockage. A more recent procedure uses a flexible metal tube (stent) that is inserted into the blockage and released to expand and hold the artery open. They even have stents that are coated with various medications.

There are complications with each of these procedures but, in general, heart pain is relieved, heart function is improved, and patients generally experience improved quality of life for a while. In some patients, these procedures have extended life when compared to people who opt not to have the procedures.

There is a downside to these treatments, however. Eating a poor American diet can plug arteries that supply blood to the heart, but what about the other arteries in the body? Don't the same disease processes that cause artery disease in vessels of the heart also affect arteries in other parts of the body? The "fix me up, Doc" mentality supposes that once a procedure has been completed, the problem will go away, when in fact, the procedure only "fixed" a blockage at one site.

Cardiovascular disease is a systemic disease; this means that it affects the entire vascular system, not just the vessels of the heart, but also arteries in the neck and brain (a leading cause of strokes). It is estimated that 2% of the population aged 40–60 years and 6% of adults older than 70 years have arteries in their arms and legs that are partially blocked, causing muscles to be starved for oxygen.[29] This is a painful condition called claudication.

Suppose you have a blocked artery in your heart and you have a bypass procedure. Are you cured? Of the veins that are used to bypass plugged arteries, 30–50% become plugged again after five to seven years.[30] That's right. You spend $65,000 for bypass surgery, you have relatively clean veins from your own body grafted into your plugged arteries, and approximately half of these clean bypass veins will get plugged up again after five to seven years.

Did the problem go away? Well, maybe for a little while. What if you had the balloon procedure on your blocked artery? After just four to six months, 30–50% of the ballooned arteries reclose.[31] When this occurs, bypass surgery or angioplasty is often repeated. Even 20–30% of arteries that have been propped open with a stent can become plugged again— that's why they try coating them with various medications.[32]

Despite the fantastic technology used in treating cardiovascular disease, the "fix me up, Doc" attitude is short sighted.[33] The problem (heart disease) may have been temporarily addressed, but the cause (an unhealthy lifestyle) remains and will continue to cause vessel disease unless it is changed. The most sophisticated medical procedures in the world are designed to treat disease; this book is about helping you prevent diseases before they can cause pain, suffering, and premature death.

Despite all that we know about good health, the medical community is almost exclusively designed to treat, not prevent, chronic diseases.

Doctor Knows Best

When teaching students and talking to adults, there is one question that always gets asked: "If good nutrition and regular physical activity are so important, how come my doctor has never asked me about my lifestyle habits?" This is a great question because it generally begins a discussion about the current state of disease prevention in the United States. First of all, physicians do care about your health; they have spent their adult lives becoming skilled medical practitioners. But despite all that we know about good health, the medical community is almost exclusively designed to treat, not prevent, chronic diseases.

In a national survey of 13,000 obese adults who had recently had a routine medical exam, only 42% of them were counseled by their physicians to lose weight.[34] If physicians don't suggest weight loss for obese patients, what about those who are just overweight? Regarding exercise, only 35% of adults report that their physician mentioned regular exercise as an important part of good health and, for most of those, it was mentioned only as a treatment for some already existing health problem.[35]

Have you ever gone to see your doctor because you were feeling great? Probably not. We typically go see a doctor when there is something wrong. The term we use to refer to personal medical attention is *health care*, but that really isn't an accurate description. Medical care in the United States is really "disease" care; we seek medical attention when we have diseases or problems.

As mentioned earlier, your "disease" care provider is expertly trained in diagnosing and treating all manner of diseases and ailments. They do some early detection activities, like breast and colon exams, but these are early detection efforts, not prevention. The current medical model in the United States is a treatment-oriented approach. Physicians are not required to take any nutrition or physical activity instruction in medical school; how could they? It takes years just to learn how to do the medical procedures that currently exist. Chances are a local dietitian or exercise physiologist will know far more about good nutrition and physical activity than your physician, but you can be sure your physician understands diseases better than anyone.

All of this is complicated. Insurance will not pay a physician to talk to you about your nutrition or physical activity. Insurance pays for medications, procedures, surgery, and clinical testing, but not in-depth patient counseling. And because doctors don't get paid for talking with their patients about healthy lifestyles, few do it.

There are several other reasons doctors don't counsel their patients on these risks. Most have never read the information you are reading in this book; there is simply too much for them to keep up with as it is. They don't know about this research. Perhaps the biggest reason doctors don't talk about healthy lifestyles with their patients is because they don't believe patients will do anything anyway. Why waste time talking about good nutrition and physical activity if the patient is unlikely to make the necessary behavior changes?

Even presidents don't practice prevention

The disease treatment focus of our medical system was never so obvious than when former President Bill Clinton had bypass surgery. The president of the United States has better medical care and attention than anyone on the planet. Three and a half years after leaving office, Clinton experienced mild chest pain and tightness. Medical tests revealed that four of the main arteries in his heart were almost entirely blocked. Most people with that much blockage have a major heart attack or suffer sudden death. Within a couple days he underwent quadruple bypass, which rerouted blood around the four blocked arteries. How could this much blockage be found in a person who has had the best medical care in the world? The medical system failed to keep the former president healthy because the system is not designed to prevent disease. Clinton had high cholesterol, a fondness for junk food, and occasional weight problems. These three risk factors are most likely to blame for his condition. His medical care did exactly what it is designed to do: treat medical problems when they occur. A better, healthier approach would have been to help him first change his lifestyle, then medicate if necessary and treat when needed. A healthy lifestyle would have helped keep his arteries clean and may have prevented his surgery.

Unfortunately, there is some truth to this. There is a lot of I-don't-care-itis out there. So, if patients won't change lifestyles, the next best thing is to prescribe medications. After all, it is much easier to take a pill than it is to walk every day or eat a healthy diet. Apparently, even this is still asking too much of patients: on average patients take their medications only half the time.[36] Whether people are trying to adhere to a new lifestyle or a new medication, human behavior is hard to change, and compliance is never perfect.

In the future it is possible that the health care industry may be more like the dental industry. Dentists have been pushing dental hygiene with regular brushing and flossing, which prevent tooth decay and help people avoid future dental work. A dentist's first line of treatment is prevention. If you still need dental care, they also provide great treatment, but the focus is on preventing dental diseases before they happen.

If a kitchen sink is backed up and the water is running over the edge of the sink onto the floor, one solution is to keep mopping up the floor as the water continues to spill. This is like our current medical system. Another solution would be to turn off the water at the tap (the source of the water) to prevent the water from spilling over. Someday we may have a medical system that works like the dental industry—prevent first, then treat.

POINTS TO REMEMBER

- Think long term when you think about your health. Small investments in good nutrition and physical activity now will have a big payoff in the future.

- Many chronic diseases get started early in life. The sooner you adopt a healthy lifestyle, the sooner you can begin preventing disease.

- Our American or Western lifestyle is a main cause of chronic disease in the United States.

- Commit to good nutrition, and you'll get the upper hand in avoiding cancer. With your good example, your children will also learn to eat healthy foods, be active, and avoid many of the diseases that adults experience.

4

Where Are You?

Happiness is nothing more than good health and a bad memory.
—Albert Schweitzer (1875–1965)

A YOUNG WOMAN WE'LL CALL KAREN started working as a pediatric nurse at a hospital in Philadelphia in 1980. Her professional training prepared her for a career in which she could practice medicine and help children. Besides her medical training, she also had a personal interest in her own health and tried to take care of her body.

Even before 1980, researchers had begun to document the importance of good nutrition and physical activity. Karen didn't eat a lot of red meat; ate plenty of fruits, vegetables, and whole grains; exercised every day; didn't smoke; and maintained a healthy body weight. Little did she know when she started her career that she would become part of one of the largest studies of health ever conducted.

In 1976, the National Institutes of Health agreed to fund a cohort study of 122,000 nurses.[1] Researchers recruited nurses to participate in the study and during the first year and every other year thereafter, these nurses made their personal health, and medical information available to researchers, who agreed to keep the information confidential. This study continues today.

In 1994, 14 years after the study started, researchers looked at what was happening to the nurses' health. They determined how many of the nurses had died of coronary heart disease; then they put the nurses' health data into groups in order to answer specific questions. For example, was there a difference in the number of deaths between nurses who were obese versus nurses who were not obese? The data was divided according to many different factors, including diet, exercise, tobacco use, body weight, and alcohol consumption.

In one analysis, researchers used this data to determine how many of the heart disease deaths that occurred in the first 14 years were related to lifestyle behaviors. The number of deaths among exercisers was much lower than for non-exercisers; those who ate cereal with fiber and little saturated fat and trans fat had fewer deaths than those who did not. Those in the group that avoided tobacco had fewer deaths, and those in the group that drank limited amounts of alcohol appeared to have some protection.

What about nurses who worked hard to have good health and did everything right—those who didn't smoke, kept a healthy weight, ate a good diet, exercised, and drank only a moderate amount of alcohol? Karen was in this group, which represented a relatively small portion of all the nurses—only 3%. When nurses without these healthy lifestyles were followed over time, they showed rates of heart disease death that were six times greater than those among nurses who had lived like Karen.

By studying large groups of women like Karen, researchers have shown that 82% of coronary deaths in women are related to individual health behaviors. These results also indicate that death due to heart disease is rarely caused by an inherited gene or an act of God; it means most cases of heart disease are preventable, and most deaths from this disease are premature.

Twenty years before the Nurses' Health Study, the Framingham Heart Study,[2] the first large-scale study of heart disease, began to identify the major pieces of the health puzzle. (See chapter 2.) There are several well-known pieces to the puzzle, and most Americans can probably identify many of them: high blood pressure, tobacco use, high blood cholesterol, and excessive body weight.

If you are overweight or a tobacco user, it's obvious you have an in-creased health risk. But unless you've had your blood pressure and choles-terol measured, there is no way of knowing if these are high and therefore put you at risk because there are no symptoms. If you don't know what your health risks are, efforts to improve health are unlikely to happen. What is your current diet? Do you get enough exercise? Karen had a healthy lifestyle, and, though we don't know what her blood pressure and cholesterol were, she was already doing the right things.

Many of you who are reading this book may already work hard to eat right and exercise. If you have your blood pressure and cholesterol checked and they still indicate an increased risk, maybe it's time to visit with your physician about starting on a medication to help you lower your risk. The next section includes some simple self-evaluations to help you measure your current lifestyle and identify your health risks. They will help you identify what you are doing right and what might need some attention.

Assess Yourself

This is really easy. Think about the food you ate in the last 24 hours. Count the servings of fruits, vegetables, whole grains, and red meat that you ate. A serving of fruit or vegetables is equal to a ½ cup, or about what you can fit in your cup-shaped hand or a single whole fruit or vegetable. A serving of meat is about the size of a deck of cards or a single hamburger patty. A serving of whole grains is one piece of whole-grain bread or a cup of whole-grain cereal. How many servings in each category did you get in the last 24 hours? Do the last 24 hours represent approximately the way you eat every day of the week? To see how your diet is right now, answer the following questions:

Over the past week, what was your average number of fruit servings per day?　　＿＿＿＿

Over the past week, what was your average number of vegetable servings per day?　＿＿＿＿

Total ＿＿＿＿

If your total is greater than five, you are doing great (more is even better).

Last week, what was your average number of whole grain servings per day?
(This includes whole-grain cereals, bread, rice, and pasta.)　　＿＿＿＿

You should strive for at least six servings of grains per day and at least half of these should be whole grains.

How many servings of red meat did you eat last week?　　＿＿＿＿

The best evidence we have so far indicates red meat should be eaten sparingly, one to two servings per week.

How many days in a typical week do you accumulate 30 minutes of moderate-intensity physical activity?　　＿＿＿＿

To get the benefits associated with being physically active, you should accumulate 30 minutes of moderate-intensity physical activity most days of the week.

Have you ever been told by a physician that you have high blood pressure?
Yes _____ No _____ Don't know _____

Systolic Blood Pressure levels[3]
<120 Normal
120–139 Early high blood pressure
140–159 High
≥160 Dangerous

Have you ever been told by a physician that you have high blood cholesterol?
Yes _____ No _____ Don't know _____

Cholesterol levels[4]
<200 Normal
200–239 Borderline high
≥240 High risk

Finally, using your height and weight, find your body mass index (BMI) in the next table; BMI is a measure of obesity risk.

Body Mass Index Chart

Height	Weight (lbs)																	
	120	130	140	150	160	170	180	190	200	210	220	230	240	250	260	270	280	>290
4'5"	30	33	35	38	40	43	45	48	50	53	55	58	60	63	65	68	70	73
4'6"	29	31	34	36	39	41	43	46	48	51	53	55	58	60	63	65	68	70
4'7"	28	30	33	35	37	40	42	44	46	49	51	53	56	58	60	63	65	67
4'8"	27	29	31	34	36	38	40	43	45	47	49	52	54	56	58	61	63	65
4'9"	26	28	30	32	35	37	39	41	43	45	48	50	52	54	56	58	61	63
4'10"	25	27	29	31	33	36	38	40	42	44	46	48	50	52	54	56	59	61
4'11"	24	26	28	30	32	34	36	38	40	42	44	46	48	50	53	55	57	59
5'0"	23	25	27	29	31	33	35	37	39	41	43	45	47	49	51	53	55	57
5'1"	23	25	26	28	30	32	34	36	38	40	42	43	45	47	49	51	53	55
5'2"	22	24	26	27	29	31	33	35	37	38	40	42	44	46	48	49	51	53
5'3"	21	23	25	27	28	30	32	34	35	37	39	41	43	44	46	48	50	51
5'4"	21	22	24	26	27	29	31	33	34	36	38	39	41	43	45	46	48	50
5'5"	20	22	23	25	27	28	30	32	33	35	37	38	40	42	43	45	47	48
5'6"	19	21	23	24	26	27	29	31	32	34	36	37	39	40	42	44	45	47
5'7"	19	20	22	23	25	27	28	30	31	33	34	36	38	39	41	42	44	45
5'8"	18	20	21	23	24	26	27	29	30	32	33	35	36	38	40	41	43	44
5'9"	18	19	21	22	24	25	27	28	30	31	32	34	35	37	38	40	41	43
5'10"	17	19	20	22	23	24	26	27	29	30	32	33	34	36	37	39	40	42
5'11"	17	18	20	21	22	24	25	26	28	29	31	32	33	35	36	38	39	40
6'0"	16	18	19	20	22	23	24	26	27	28	30	31	33	34	35	37	38	39
6'1"	16	17	18	20	21	22	24	25	26	28	29	30	32	33	34	36	37	38
6'2"	15	17	18	19	21	22	23	24	26	27	28	30	31	32	33	35	36	37
6'3"	15	16	17	19	20	21	22	24	25	26	27	29	30	31	32	34	35	36
6'4"	15	16	17	18	19	21	22	23	24	26	27	28	29	30	32	33	34	35
6'5"	14	15	17	18	19	20	21	23	24	25	26	27	28	30	31	32	33	34
6'6"	14	15	16	17	18	20	21	22	23	24	25	27	28	29	30	31	32	34
6'7"	14	15	16	17	18	19	20	21	23	24	25	26	27	28	29	30	32	33
6'8"	13	14	15	16	18	19	20	21	22	23	24	25	26	27	29	30	31	32
6'9"	13	14	15	16	17	18	19	20	21	23	24	25	26	27	28	29	30	31
6'10"	13	14	15	16	17	18	19	20	21	22	23	24	25	26	27	28	29	30

Underweight   Ideal weight   Overweight   Obese
                     (low risk)   (moderate risk)   (high risk)

What is your Body Mass Index? _____

Body Mass Index Categories[5]
<19	Underweight
19–24	Ideal weight, low risk
25–29	Overweight, moderate risk
≥30	Obese, high risk

Health Risks Vary

If you have one or more of these health risks, you are not doomed to poor health; almost everyone has some health risks. Suppose you have gained weight over the years, and now, according to your BMI score, you are in the obese category.

Researchers have gathered together the best information available and have drawn a line in the sand—that line is a BMI of 30. If your BMI is 30 or more, your risk of premature death and disease is significant. But that line is somewhat arbitrary. Figure 4.1 shows the risk of premature death and disease according to body weight. With the BMI category you just calculated, find your weight category in the next figure and look at the segment of the curved line above your category.

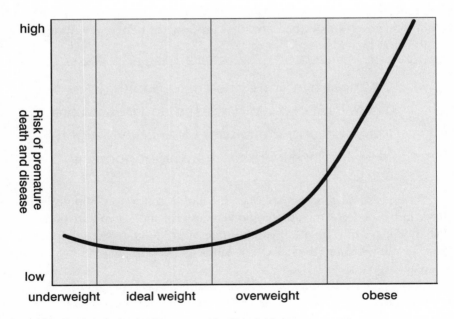

Figure 4.1 Premature death, disease, and body weight

The risk of premature death increases as weight increases, while the fewest chronic diseases and deaths are found among those with ideal body weight. As weight increases, the risk of disease increases slowly at first, but as weight continues to increase, the curve becomes steeper and steeper and risk increases more dramatically. Having a BMI of 30 simply means a person's risk is significant because the curve becomes steeper and steeper after that point. The figure also illustrates that there is some risk even for those who are simply overweight. Even though obesity is defined as having a BMI of 30 or greater, health risks begin to increase as weight goes above ideal weight.

Excess body weight is not the only health risk that follows this type of curve. Just as researchers have drawn a line in the sand for obesity, similar lines exist for cholesterol and blood pressure, and health risks are higher for anyone who is not in the healthy or normal ranges. High blood cholesterol is the best predictor of heart disease that we currently have. Blood cholesterol levels less than 200 are considered healthy. As cholesterol levels increase, the risk increases slowly at first, then becomes steadily higher and higher as cholesterol increases. If you were to replace the labels on the bottom of Figure 4.1 with "normal," "borderline high," and "high" in reference to blood cholesterol and plot the death and disease data associated with cholesterol, the resulting curve would look almost exactly the same. The same is true for blood pressure. The risk associated with having high blood pressure is small when pressures are low, but it increases dramatically as pressures increase.

Almost everyone has some health risks.
The fewest chronic diseases and deaths are
found among those with ideal body weight.
Health risks increase as weight goes up.

There is some good news hidden in all of this, however. Suppose you have high blood pressure, high blood cholesterol, and/or you are obese. What happens to your risk if you improve your lifestyle? You will lower your health risks, and the risk curve will begin working in your favor rather than against you.

Just as the probability of early death and disease goes up dramatically as risks increase, the opposite is true when you lower health risks. The higher the risk in the beginning, the further the risk decreases, and the more improvement in health is available. People just like you and I can and do change behaviors, and when they do, good things happen—and I've got proof.

A few years ago, researchers from Rockford, Illinois, and I convinced six large corporations to help their employees improve their lifestyles. Four hundred and forty-two employees participated in a video-based program designed to help them eat better and get regular exercise. After eight weeks, high blood pressures among employees were reduced by an average of 10 points and those with high blood cholesterol saw an average decrease of 13%. In six weeks, the men lost 12 pounds on average and the women lost 8 pounds on average.[6] All these changes occurred just by changing their diets and exercising.

We realized that the design of our study could not provide proof that changing lifestyles could improve health, so we applied for and received a large grant to conduct a randomized clinical trial to test a program designed to help individuals improve their nutrition and physical activity habits.[7] We recruited 377 people to participate in our trial, and after just eight weeks, the participants dramatically improved their physical activity; consumed significantly more fruits, vegetables, and whole grains; and reduced the amount of meat they consumed. Those who started with high blood pressure saw their diastolic blood pressure drop by seven points on average, and those with initially high blood cholesterol experienced an average reduction of 12%.

Eight weeks is not a very long time, so we continued to follow and evaluate what happened to these people after six months. After six months, participants not only continued eating more fruits, vegetables, and whole grains than they did before, but they actually increased the amount of good foods they were eating.

Typically, after people change behaviors, many slowly revert back to their old ways of eating and sometimes stop exercising. But in this study, even after six months, good nutrition and physical activity were still increasing. Participants continued to lose weight, blood pressures were significantly lowered, instances of diabetes decreased, and those who had high blood cholesterol saw their cholesterol improve after six weeks and stay that way for at least six months. The average age of our participants was 50! Who says you can't teach an old dog new tricks!

When people learn *why* they should change lifestyles, they can make significant changes in diet and physical activity, and they can dramatically reduce their risks for cardiovascular disease, cancer, diabetes, and other lifestyle-related diseases. For every 1% drop in total cholesterol, the risk of having a heart attack drops by 2–3%; and for every one-point drop in elevated diastolic blood pressure, there is another 2–3% drop in heart attack risk.[8]

This may not seem like much, but taken together, health can take dramatic turns for the better. For our study participants, the average improvements in blood cholesterol and blood pressure translated into a 38–57% reduction in the risk of heart disease. These individuals cut their risk of heart attack in half by adopting a healthy diet and spending more time getting physical activity with spouses, friends, and family members.

But these results were based on individuals who already had elevated blood pressure and cholesterol. What about people who don't have health risks but also don't have a healthy lifestyle? You know these people—they eat whatever they want, may not exercise, and still feel fine. When these low-risk but unhealthy people adopt a healthy lifestyle, their blood pressure and cholesterol get even better.

The Dose Response

What health benefits can come to someone who is just starting to exercise? *Dose response* is a term that describes how a small dose of a drug can have a substantial impact, but the more of a drug you take, the less impact there is (no additional reduction of pain, for example). A single dose makes a big difference; a huge dose is only slightly better but more dangerous. The same principle also applies to exercise.

Suppose you have a sprained ankle. It hurts, so you take a couple aspirin to help reduce the pain. The two aspirin you took will alleviate most of the pain. What happens to the rest of the pain if you take more aspirin? The first two pills reduced about as much of the pain as can be reduced with aspirin. No matter how many more pills you take, the amount of remaining pain will reduce only slightly, and you might overdose in the attempt.

Physical activity can be perceived as a drug to treat and prevent chronic diseases, with the dose response for physical activity similar to the dose response we see with medications. If a sedentary person becomes physically active, the health benefits are tremendous.[9,10] If that same person decides to do even more physical activity, the additional health benefits are not quite as large as with the first, smaller dose.

Karen, the nurse described at the beginning of this chapter, exercises by walking for 30–40 minutes every day. With this amount of physical activity, she is enjoying most of the benefits that are available to those who are active. Suppose she wants to be even healthier, so she decides to train for and run a marathon with a friend (in other words, take a really big dose of exercise). By participating in this additional training, her health will continue to improve, but the amount of improvement will be smaller compared to what she experienced when she went from being sedentary to walking daily.

What does this mean? A small amount of exercise is good, and a very large amount of exercise is also good, but the very large amount of exercise doesn't provide an equally large improvement in health. Who is getting the most health benefits: a person who exercises regularly every day or a person who does intense training for two hours every day? The really active person will have the most health benefits, but the overall difference between the two will be fairly small. For all the couch potatoes in the world, this is great news. If you will begin and maintain a daily exercise program, you will get a very big return on your investment—and you don't have to be a marathon runner. More on this in chapter 9.

The benefits of eating a healthy diet *do not* appear to be limited by the dose response. Most nutrition experts recommend the consumption of at least five servings of fruits or vegetables every day—"Stay Alive with Five." Others have indicated that if five is great, then nine is divine. It appears that the more you eat, the better you'll be. With fruits and vegetables there doesn't appear to be any decline in the benefits—the more you eat, the more you benefit.[11]

One Plus One Does Not Equal Two

Somewhere in America there is probably a young man who rides a motorcycle to work without a helmet. Not wearing a helmet puts some risk of premature death in his life, but not too much. He may also smoke three packs a day, never exercise, have multiple sex partners, never eat vegetables, play golf during thunderstorms, drive under the influence of alcohol, be a member of a gang, and be particularly fond of playing with explosives. Now we're talking risk. If you add up the total risk he is exposed to, you begin to see that the odds of his living a long, high-quality life are slim, but he's going to have a great time for a few years. His unfortunate premature demise is likely.

This is an extreme case of risk exposure. A more realistic example would be someone who is overweight, inactive, and has a poor diet—that includes most people in America. Being overweight will increase a person's odds of getting chronic diseases, but when we add sedentary living to this risk, the overall risk does not just double—it increases exponentially. Now, add a poor diet or any other health risk, and the odds of experiencing artery disease, cancer, or diabetes grow dramatically. The risk curve discussed earlier also applies to multiple risks except that as the number of risks increase, the curve becomes really steep, and the overall risk is large.

Doctors who treat diabetes and cardiovascular disease have identified a certain type of individual who has extremely high risk. These individuals are overweight and carry most of their excess body fat in their upper body (above the waist). They have high blood cholesterol, high blood pressure, and their bodies have trouble using insulin to keep cells supplied with energy. These people are considered to have a sinister-sounding condition called Syndrome X, sometimes called the metabolic syndrome. People with Syndrome X have several risks that are strongly associated with heart disease and diabetes.

Such a scary sounding condition should be one of those extremely uncommon medical conditions rarely seen by doctors. But it's not. Almost 30% of overweight teenagers in the United States meet the criteria for Syndrome X, and it is much worse the longer a person has a Western diet and lifestyle.[12] Seven percent of 20-year-olds have it, and 45% of all adults over age 60 have it. Women have it more than men, and African-Americans and Hispanics have higher rates than Asians and Caucasians.[13] From the 2000 census data, it is estimated that about 47 million U.S. residents have the metabolic syndrome right now—that's more than one out of every five adults.[14] This condition doesn't just happen to people; it's not like catching a cold. It starts slowly with steady increases in body weight and it is reaching epidemic proportions worldwide.

XL—eXtra Large

Do you remember your BMI score from the assessment we completed earlier? If your BMI puts you in the overweight category, you might be surprised to learn that, on average, overweight individuals die 3.2 years earlier than those who have ideal weight. Those who are obese can subtract 6.5 years from the average lifespan.[15] Obesity by itself does not cause you to die early, but excess body weight causes changes in your body, and these changes cause chronic diseases and premature death.

Six out of every ten adults in the United States today are overweight or obese.[16] Obesity among African-American women is especially high: more than half are obese and an additional 30% are overweight.[17] We are a nation of big people, and we are getting bigger every year. Our children are also gaining weight at an unprecedented rate; the best estimates available show that 15% of children are overweight or obese. The rates are especially high among Hispanics and African-Americans. Among all children, the percent who are overweight increases every year.[18] But if only 15% of children are overweight while 60% of all adults are overweight or obese, can't we assume that age causes obesity? No. It isn't age but our Western lifestyle, which is characterized by an unhealthy diet and a lack of regular physical activity.

In the United States during the past 20 years, only about 22% of adults reported getting regular physical activity and that number hasn't changed much,[19] though there may have been slight improvements in the past two years.[20] National surveys also show that the number of calories Americans consume has increased.[21] Compared to 1971, women now eat 335 more calories per day—that's equivalent to eating six Oreo cookies or one and a

---

Excess body weight does not suddenly appear; it tends to creep up on you. It is a gradual process that takes months, years, and decades. If you gain only a little weight every year, it doesn't take too many years before you become obese.

---

half bags of low-fat microwave popcorn every day. American men are eating 168 more calories each day—equal to about a 12-ounce soda. Most of these excess calories are coming from additional chips, cookies, bagels, and soda. So let's see, physical activity levels are unchanged and we are eating more. The net increase in energy in our bodies has to go somewhere. Where does it go? It is converted into fat and stored in our bodies. For the average American, weight increases slightly every year so that by the age of 65, most adults are overweight or obese.

But Americans are not the only ones who are experiencing an epidemic of obesity; every Westernized nation in the world is seeing dramatic increases in the number of adults and children who are obese. Consider Chinese who are educated and have higher incomes; they have worse lifestyles and more health risks than Chinese who are poor. In the United States, the more education and income people have, the better lifestyle they tend to have. In one country, education and income lead to poor health, and in another, they lead to good lifestyles and health.[22]

The poor in most Third World countries can be described as underfed and underweight. When most of us think of the world's poor, we think of thin, emaciated bodies. In the United States, however, undernourishment is not usually a concern among the poor. In fact, rates of obesity are highest among the American poor. These cultural ironies are linked to the level of economic development within a country and the extent to which particular parts of the population adopt a Western lifestyle. The poor in America struggle with excessive body weight, while the poor of the Third World struggle to gain weight.

Excess body weight does not suddenly appear; it tends to creep up on you. It is a gradual process that takes months, years, and decades. If you gain only a little weight every year, it doesn't take too many years before you become obese. In the United States, BMI scores for the average individual increase every year until about the age of 65, after which they tend to decline somewhat.[19]

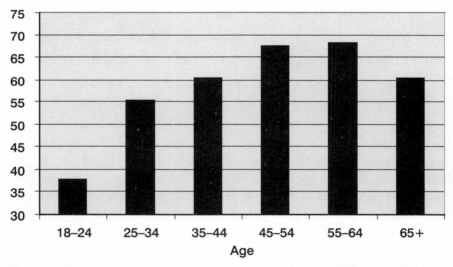

Figure 4.2 Percent of Americans who are overweight or obese according to age group[19]

The physical, financial, social, and emotional burdens associated with excessive body weight are enormous. The risk curve shown in Figure 4.1 also accurately describes other dangers associated with weight gain and obesity, not just premature death. The more body fat a person has, the higher his or her blood pressure and cholesterol become.

Overweight individuals tend to have high blood pressure and high blood cholesterol, and obese individuals tend to have even higher levels of blood pressure and cholesterol.[23,24] If blood pressure and cholesterol seem to be higher among the obese, then it stands to reason that they would also have higher rates of stroke, heart disease, and other forms of cardiovascular disease. Indeed, the obese are three times more likely to have these chronic diseases.[25-28]

Excess body fat is also associated with increased risk of certain cancers, including breast, colon, endometrial, and prostate cancers,[29-31] and a dramatic increase in the risk of gall stones and asthma.[32-34] A large study in Sweden even found that among seniors the risk of Alzheimer's disease increases 36% with every one-point increase in BMI.[35] Worst of all, excessive body weight is directly related to diabetes.

Using the most accurate data available,
it is estimated that 36% of all children born in the
year 2000 will be diabetic sometime in their lives;
among Hispanics, 50% will become diabetic.

There is even more scary data. The best estimates available today suggest that 7% of adults in the United States have been told by their physicians they have diabetes.[19] Diabetes is a condition in which energy (glucose) needed by the body's cells can't get into the cells. Glucose has to be escorted into cells by a hormone called insulin, but most people who have diabetes have cells that no longer recognize insulin and don't let glucose enter. The glucose backs up in the bloodstream and, without proper medical treatment and adoption of healthy lifestyles, organs are damaged. It is a lot like being at the gas station with an empty gas tank. You are at the fuel pump, but you can't open the lid of the tank. As a result, your car is starving for fuel while the fuel is just out of reach.

Diabetics develop complications with their hearts, nerves, feet, eyes, and kidneys, and they are three times more likely to have heart disease and strokes.[36] Because diabetes is directly related to body mass index and how much upper body fat a person has, the recent increase in obesity among Americans is an ominous sign for the future.[37,38]

Using the most accurate data available, it is estimated that 36% of all children born in the year 2000 will be diabetic sometime in their lives; among Hispanics, 50% will become diabetic.[39] Such a dramatic increase in the number of individuals with diabetes will be America's most pressing public health issue. Diabetes associated with excessive body weight used to be found only in adults; in fact, it used to be called adult onset diabetes. Today, pediatricians now regularly see this type of diabetes in sedentary, overweight children. It is entirely possible that diabetes will shorten life so much that many parents will outlive their children.

Taking Back Control

It is a little overwhelming and somewhat depressing to think of the magnitude of these lifestyle-related health issues. It would be even worse if there was nothing anyone could do about it—but there is. A few years ago, physicians who treat and study diabetes tried a bold experiment. They recruited patients who were considered pre-diabetic (they weren't considered to be diabetic yet, but probably would be with more time). Some of the study participants took a diabetes medication, some of them participated in a lifestyle modification program, and some took a placebo pill.[40] The researchers planned on following the participants for five years and hoped to see a difference in that time.

After two and a half years, the federal government ended the study. Many of the participants who were taking the placebo had become diabetic, while the healthy lifestyle group had less than half as many new cases of diabetes. The medication also had some effect, but it was not nearly as powerful as the effect of a good diet and regular physical activity. The medication also had substantial side effects. A similar study was completed in Finland and found the same results.[41] Both of these studies show that despite the disease burden that awaits many overweight Americans, health can improve and adoption of a healthy lifestyle can change the future.

Individuals who adopt healthy lifestyles can improve all aspects of Syndrome X.[42] Diabetics who engage in a walking program can significantly reduce their risk of cardiovascular death.[43] Adults who adopt healthy lifestyles and lose weight reduce many cancer and cardiovascular disease risk factors. In short, most chronic diseases and weight gain in the United States can be prevented with a healthy lifestyle. Not everyone has the same level of motivation and commitment as nurse Karen, but everyone does have the ability to be healthy if they make small but steady lifestyle improvements.

POINTS TO REMEMBER

- The likelihood of getting chronic diseases and experiencing early death increases as your health risks increase.

- There is hope. If you lower your health risks by changing your lifestyle and heeding the advice of your doctor, you will reduce your risk of disease and early death.

- The increasing rate of overweight and obese people is America's number one health problem. If you want to control your weight, you need to change your lifestyle.

PART TWO

What

CHAPTER 5

Food in Its Original Form

In all things of nature there is something of the marvelous.
—Aristotle

POPCORN IS PRETTY COOL WHEN YOU THINK ABOUT IT. You take a small kernel of corn, heat it up to just the right temperature, and in just a few seconds . . . BANG! The kernel explodes, turning itself inside out and into a bizarre shape that is 45 times larger than its original size.

A popcorn kernel, like every type of cereal grain has three distinct parts: the shell, also called the fiber or bran; the inner starch or flour; and the germ. The germ, or embryo, is the part of the seed that grows into a new plant. A popcorn kernel is almost perfectly round; has a hard, airtight shell; and, most important, the starch inside the shell has just the right amount of moisture.

When popcorn is heated, the starch gets very hot, and the moisture inside starts to turn to steam. Additional heat creates more steam, and the pressure builds until the shell can no longer withstand the pressure and explodes—and the superheated starch expands into space. Add salt, a little butter, and—presto!—you are ready to enjoy a healthy, whole-grain treat.

It is whole grain because it contains the *whole* grain, everything—the fibrous bran, the germ, and the starch. Next time you eat popcorn, take a good look at what you are eating. The most obvious part is the white fluffy starch. It is soft to chew and has a nutty flavor. Tucked deep inside the fluffy part you will see what is left of the shell. The little fragments still sticking to the starch are all that is left of a shell that did its best to withstand the pressure. If you popped the corn in the microwave, some of the shell fragments may still be in the bag or the container along with those dreaded "grannies"—you know, the kernels that didn't pop. They didn't pop because either the moisture content was slightly off or the shell leaked and the pressure escaped.

Take a good look at a granny. Every kernel of corn has a point. That point is the location of the germ. When you eat popcorn, you are eating everything the grain has to offer, the whole grain. Other whole grains, such as oatmeal, wheat, barley, buckwheat, millet, and rye, are just a few of the many different grains grown as food. Figure 5.1 shows the parts of a kernel of wheat. Just like popcorn, there is the outer covering, or bran; the inner starch, or flour; and the germ. It looks a little different, but all the required parts are there.

If you take some kernels of wheat and grind them into powder, you get whole wheat flour. Unfortunately, the flour many of us are accustomed to comes from wheat that has been ground and separated into something very different from whole wheat flour. This kind of flour is made by milling wheat kernels until they are flattened, and then sending the flattened grain through a series of screens and rollers until the bran and germ are removed, leaving just bleached, white, refined flour. (For every 100 pounds of whole

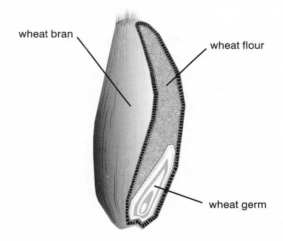

wheat bran

wheat flour

wheat germ

Figure 5.1 A kernel of wheat

wheat that goes in, only 72 pounds comes out as flour, and most of the parts that are removed during this process are used for cattle feed.) Malted barley, bleaching agents, and enrichments are added to the final flour before it is packaged.

The resulting refined, bleached, white flour has a unique taste, texture, and baking quality. White flour has become as American as apple pie. It is the primary source of energy for a hungry nation, and it is the main ingredient for most breads and flour-based foods. In fact, it permeates all segments of our food supply: noodles, pasta, white bread, pancakes, bagels, doughnuts, many prepackaged foods like cold cereals, and most prepared baked foods like muffins and cakes.

Historically, refined white flour was so expensive that only the wealthy were able to afford and consume it; the poor continued to use whole wheat flour. Today economically affluent Western nations have been able to reduce the cost of producing white flour to the point that even the poor can eat foods made from bleached white flour. Historically, a diet based on white flour did not seem to be a reason for concern, but in the last 20 years, large studies from all over the world have revealed that diets based on products made from refined flour and starches are not ideal. Some nutrition extremists have even been known to proclaim, "The whiter the bread, the sooner you're dead."

Refined flour and starches are not white poison, nor are they considered to be anywhere near as bad as something like smoking. But as un-American as it may sound, individuals who have diets composed mostly of products made from white flour and refined starches are at a significant health disadvantage. They have an increased risk of many chronic diseases because although these foods do not cause disease, they fail to prevent disease. Eating whole grains provides a level of protection that is no longer available once the grain has been turned into white flour.

"Food in its original form" refers to food that is close to its natural state; highly processed and refined foods are no longer in their natural state. Some may be close to their original form (whole wheat flour), while others give you no hint of their origin. It might be hard to tell what a Hostess Twinkie is made of, but in its original form, a Twinkie is made from wheat. The further a food gets from its original form, the less health benefits it has. I don't know of anyone who died by eating Twinkies, but as you will learn in this chapter, the closer your foods are to their original form, the better off you will be.

Sunday Dinner

Besides grains, other starchy foods are often altered before they arrive on the dinner table. Brown rice is refined and stripped of it fibrous covering to become white rice; potatoes are skinned, boiled, and mashed to become mashed potatoes. These are refining processes that alter the food from its natural form. I realize that putting white rice and mashed potatoes on the unhealthy food hit list is unpatriotic—even traitorous—and might bring on a flood of hate mail. I beg for your patience and understanding, at least until you have finished this chapter; then you can send the hate mail.

You should know that I still eat white rice and mashed potatoes. I also eat meat, but not very much or very often. Every week our family will join together for a nice Sunday dinner. The typical dinner might include fresh corn, peas, carrots, and onions that have been baked in the oven over a small, lean beef roast, sometimes mashed potatoes might be prepared, and all of this served with a little gravy. The mashed potatoes and the meat occupy only a small portion of the plates, which are already loaded with corn, peas, carrots, and onions. The mashed potatoes and meat are delicious, but they are not the main course.

Likewise, white rice might be prepared and served with stir-fried vegetables. Our other meals of the day include whole-grain breads, oatmeal, whole-grain cold cereals for breakfast, and even whole-grain pastas. I hope you are beginning to realize that there are very few foods that should be avoided. There are some that should be eaten every day, but in moderation, and lots of great foods that should be eaten at most meals.

Remember the Healthy Eating Pyramid from chapter 1? It's shown again on the next page. The bottom and middle portions of the pyramid show the great foods—whole grains, plant oils, nuts, legumes, and fruits and vegetables—that should be eaten every day. The upper portions show fish, poultry, eggs, and dairy that should be eaten almost every day, and the top shows those foods that should be eaten sparingly. Notice that white rice, mashed potatoes, and red meat are on the top, along with butter, white bread, pasta, and sweets.

The Healthy Eating Pyramid was developed by researchers at the Harvard School of Public Health after an exhaustive review of every nutrition study. It represents the best information we have right now—it is not done yet, and as more science is completed, there will undoubtedly be a few more changes. What is important is that the pyramid is driven by the science, not special interest groups or lobbyists from the meat or dairy industries. The science behind the pyramid and the need to eat more whole grains is striking. Let's look at some of the evidence.

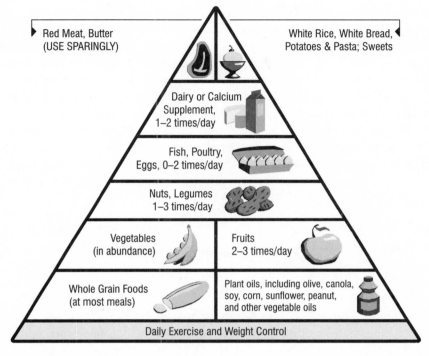

Red Meat, Butter
(USE SPARINGLY)

White Rice, White Bread,
Potatoes & Pasta; Sweets

Dairy or Calcium
Supplement,
1–2 times/day

Fish, Poultry,
Eggs, 0–2 times/day

Nuts, Legumes
1–3 times/day

Vegetables
(in abundance)

Fruits
2–3 times/day

Whole Grain Foods
(at most meals)

Plant oils, including olive, canola,
soy, corn, sunflower, peanut,
and other vegetable oils

Daily Exercise and Weight Control

Figure 5.2 Healthy Eating Pyramid. Adapted from www.hsph.harvard.edu/nutritionsource

Why You Should Care about Whole Grains

The Healthy Eating Pyramid recommends that we eat whole grains at most meals. One serving of whole grains equals one piece of whole-grain bread or one cup of whole-grain cereal. That doesn't seem like a lot, does it? But if you're like most Americans, you eat less than one serving of whole grains per day.[1] In fact, only 13% of Americans eat at least one serving per day.[2] Since studies have demonstrated that there are health benefits to those who eat at least one serving of whole grains each day, I'm guessing most people either don't know about these studies or they don't care.

There are other reasons why so many Americans fail to eat whole grains and fail to receive the health benefits. Only about 5% of American foods that contain wheat or oats actually contain whole grains. This means that whole-grain foods are not readily available, but this is likely a reflection of consumer demand; consumers prefer refined flour, and food manufacturers are eager to keep the consumer happy.

The most common complaint reported by those who eat white refined flour is constipation. Since the flour no longer contains much fiber, the digested flour doesn't hold much water and tends to move very slowly through the large intestine. In some cases, hemorrhoids can result from the "pushing" needed to move the stool along every time a person has a bowel movement. As uncomfortable as constipation and hemorrhoids are, however, they aren't the real impact that lack of whole grains can have on health.

Many large cohort studies have studied the effects of whole grains on quality of life, chronic disease, and even premature death.[2,3] It is hard to imagine how whole grains might extend life or even prevent heart disease or certain cancers, but they do. Ten different cohort studies that looked at

---

For every 10 grams of fiber you average per day, your risk of heart attack goes down 14% and your risk of heart disease death goes down 27%.

---

whole grains have been completed in the United States and Europe.[4] When taken together, these studies followed a quarter of a million women and almost 100,000 men for up to 10 years. All but one of these studies showed that the more dietary fiber people eat, the lower their risk of heart disease.[5]

For every 10 grams of fiber you average per day, your risk of heart attack goes down 14% and your risk of heart disease death goes down 27%.[4] Just during breakfast you could get 10 grams of fiber if you consumed the right foods. Say you ate just two slices of whole-grain bread or a cup of whole-grain cold cereal like Cheerios; you would consume 10 grams of fiber! These are just two examples of high-fiber foods. There are many whole grains, fruits, and vegetables that contain fiber, and all help protect against heart disease and heart disease death if you eat them. Another large study showed that just by eating whole-grain breakfast cereals, you can significantly reduce your heart disease risk—by 35%.[6]

Over 45 studies have looked at the connection between whole grains and cancer.[7] Imagine nerdy scientists all over the world gathering nutrition information from all kinds of people, asking all kinds of health-related questions, and then spending years analyzing and publishing all the results in scientific journals where other nerdy scientists can critique what was done. All these studies used different research methods and different ways of measuring nutrition. Amazingly, only 3 of the 45 studies failed to show that eating whole grains prevented certain cancers. The cancers studied included breast, ovarian, colorectal, pancreatic, stomach, and other cancers.

You will recall from chapter 4 that the number of individuals with diabetes is rapidly growing, and, unless things change, most of today's children will be tomorrow's diabetics. Whole grains can protect against diabetes.

Consider refined flour and whole-grain wheat flour. Which one do you think is digested more quickly? Refined flour reaches the bloodstream quickly and causes a dramatic increase in insulin.[8] Whole grains, on the other hand, cause only a small, slow increase in insulin because the energy in whole grains takes longer to reach the bloodstream. Those who eat more than two servings of whole-grain foods a day don't have nearly the amount of circulating insu-

---

Individuals who have diets composed mostly of white flour and refined starches are at a significant health disadvantage.

---

lin and are also 30% less likely to get diabetes in comparison to those who eat few whole-grain foods during the day.[9-11] As with heart disease, those who eat whole-grain cereals seem to get a large level of protection from them.

Some really clever scientists also looked at whole-grain diets and the risk of having a stroke.[12] Among 75,000 women, those who ate two or more servings of whole grains were 36% less likely to have a stroke than those who ate few whole grains. A study was completed in 2000 that looked at death rates in people who ate refined flour versus those who ate whole grains.[13] Compared to women with diets that included refined flour, women with diets of whole-grain foods had a 17% lower death rate. Maybe there really is something to the saying, "The whiter the bread, the sooner you're dead!"

How can this be? How can refined flour be responsible for these increases in disease and premature death? I try not to think of it in this way; rather, I like to think that foods that are made from refined flour just don't contribute to my good health. They fill me up, but they don't give me any protection or extra benefit; it is as if they are "health neutral." The way the body reacts to refined flour is different than its response to whole grains.

What's Going on Here?

If whole grains can provide so much protection against so many different diseases, what makes them so special? Grains are plants and plants have been around for a long time, struggling to reproduce, trying to stay alive, and doing their best to avoid diseases, bacteria, fungi, ultraviolet light, viruses, and other threats to their existence. In their struggle for survival, they have developed specialized defenses.

Plants naturally produce a variety of chemicals called phytochemicals (the word *phyto* means "plant"). I like to think of them as "fight-o-chemicals" because they have the ability to fight off attackers. Some of these phytochemicals can kill harmful bacteria and viruses, some can kill fungus, and others protect the plant from the harmful rays of the sun. There are many different kinds of phytochemicals, but for now it is important to understand that they are found in all plants, including whole grains.

You will recall that the milling process that is used with whole grains strips away the outer bran and the germ. The bran and germ contain high amounts of fiber, vitamins, minerals, some protein, and phytochemicals. The center portion of the grain, the flour, is almost all carbohydrates, with just a few vitamins. So where did all the phytochemicals and fiber in the grain end up? Do you remember those cattle and horses that get the bran and germ left over after the milling process? Well, they must be the healthiest critters in the country!

I can't help but wonder if our cattle have really low rates of cow strokes, cow heart attacks, cow cancer, and even cow constipation. Unfortunately, most of what makes up the "whole" (the fiber, vitamins, minerals, protein, and phytochemicals) found in the original *whole* grain ends up being fed to cows instead of to your kids.

Even though whole grains have been shown to be healthy, our understanding of how they protect us from disease and premature death is limited. There are, however, several possible explanations. The first involves the phytochemicals that are so predominant in whole grains. Phytochemicals are known to be associated with the prevention and treatment of four of the leading causes of death in the United States—cancer, diabetes, cardiovascular disease, and hypertension.[14] They are involved in all sorts of metabolic processes that occur in the body. They can also help prevent cancer cell replication, prevent cell damage, and even decrease cholesterol levels.

Whole grains also contain fiber, which is nothing more than a complicated sugar molecule called a complex carbohydrate. Wood is a form of fiber, and if you've ever burned wood, you know that energy is released when it's burned. But unless you're a beaver or a termite, eating wood won't give you much energy because you lack the enzymes needed to break down the wood into usable sugars.

Whole grains and fruits and vegetables contain several different types of fiber. Some of it is like wood in that it is nondigestible. Corn, peas, cabbage, cauliflower, and bran from grains contain fiber that is nondigestible. These foods end up passing through your intestines in just about the same form they were in when they were eaten. Though it may seem that the food wasn't of much value to you because it wasn't digested, your body still receives a benefit by having it.

If you've ever made oatmeal or another hot breakfast cereal, you know you have to add a lot of water when you cook it because the grains

Will the real wheat bread please stand up?

As you are looking at the different grain products at your local store, don't be deceived by many of the food manufacturer's marketing ploys. If you see bread that says "wheat bread" or "stone-ground wheat bread" on the label, you might want to look a little closer. The only guarantee you have that the bread you are looking at is actually whole grain is if it lists whole wheat as the first ingredient.

The ingredients list is required by law to be accurate; if the main ingredient is whole wheat flour, you will be getting whole wheat flour—all the good stuff. If, however, you see that the main ingredient is wheat flour, enriched wheat flour, or flour, you should read on because you will also likely see another ingredient called caramel color. If you were to look at a slice of this bread, you will see that it looks dark like whole wheat bread, and it might smell like whole wheat bread, and the package it came from probably says wheat on it, but don't be fooled— it's not made of whole wheat. It is baked with refined white flour and made to look like whole wheat bread by adding caramel coloring. Here is a typical "fake" whole wheat bread ingredient list; notice the flour and caramel coloring.

INGREDIENTS
ENRICHED FLOUR (FLOUR, BARLEY MALT, NIACIN, IRON, THIAMINE MONONITRATE, RIBOFLAVIN), WATER, WHOLE WHEAT FLOUR, CORN SYRUP, CONTAINS 2% OR LESS OF: YEAST, SOYBEAN OIL, WHEAT GLUTEN, SALT, DOUGH CONDITIONERS (MONO AND DIGLYCERIDES, CALCIUM AND SODIUM TEAROYL-2-LACTYLATE, CORN FLOUR, SOYA FLOUR, POTASSIUM BROMATE, ENZYMES), CALCIUM PROPIONATE (A PRESERVATIVE), YEAST NUTRIENTS (AMMONIUM SULFATE, CALCIUM SULFATE), CARAMEL COLOR, POTASSIUM SORBATE (A PRESERVATIVE)

If you wanted to really stretch the truth, you could make a food with the following ingredients, and still call it healthy wheat bread. Can you guess what it is?

INGREDIENTS
WHEAT FLOUR, TREACLE, RAW SUGAR, GLUCOSE SYRUP, WATER, PALM OIL, CITRIC ACID, MINERAL SALT, MONOGLYCERIDE, (EMULSIFIER E471), FLAVOR, ARTIFICIAL COLOR (RED 40).

It's red licorice.

absorb the water and swell to several times their original size. When you cook rice, the same thing happens. Nondigestible fiber is important because it absorbs and holds water, which makes everything pass through your digestive system more easily. Oatmeal contains both digestible and nondigestible fiber.

The ingredients in Metamucil, Fibercon, and other products designed to alleviate constipation contain cellulose, a nondigestible form of fiber that makes up cell walls in plants. Nondigestible fiber softens the stool and is believed to be associated with reduced rates of colon cancer.[15-17] Because this fiber enters the intestine undigested, it ferments; this changes the acidity of the colon and helps the body produce immune fighting cells.[14] Nondigestible fiber alters the way our bodies produce insulin, which may help us avoid diabetes, obesity, and even breast cancer.[3]

The other type of fiber in whole grains is digestible fiber (like in oatmeal). This is also found in fruits and vegetables (bananas, apples, oranges, and beans). When these foods are digested, they help control blood sugar and can lower the amount of cholesterol in the blood.[18-19] A diet that contains whole grains can prevent constipation,[20] hemorrhoids, and colon cancer, and is thought to prevent varicose veins,[21] appendicitis, and other digestive problems.[22]

How Much Whole Grains Should You Eat?

The current recommendation for eating whole grains is to make sure, whether you eat a lot of grains or a little, that half are whole grain. For example, if you typically eat six servings of grains each day, you should make sure that at least three of those servings are whole grains. Another recommendation that is easier to remember is "Three are key." Make sure you eat three servings of whole grains a day. This is easy. If you have whole-grain cereal for breakfast, whole-grain bread for lunch, and whole-grain rice or pasta at dinner, you've eaten your three servings.[3]

Despite all the scientific information that has been presented here, it is of no real value unless you accept the recommendations and make dietary changes that you can sustain for the rest of your life. Chapter 12 is devoted to helping you make those changes in your diet by giving you tips, helpful ideas, and doable goals that will enable you to change your diet and start to enjoy all the benefits that are available to those who eat well.

There is no doubt that eating whole grains provides an added level of disease protection and ultimately better health if you change your lifestyle, but the health benefits associated with whole grains only scratches the sur-

---

Why you should include whole grains (fiber) in your diet

1. It absorbs water and makes the stool softer. A soft stool makes everything pass through the digestive system a lot easier. A hard stool is part of the cause of constipation.
2. It changes the acidity in the colon, which prompts the body to produce immune fighting cells. This helps you avoid infections.
3. It alters the amount of insulin your body produces. This means the energy in whole grain foods enters the bloodstream more slowly, which helps keep your blood sugar from having wide fluctuations. (More on this in the discussion of the glycemic index in chapter 8.)
4. It contains phytochemicals, nature's health-promoting helpers.

face. Fruits and vegetables are literally packed with nutrients that are only now being identified and studied, and the results so far suggest that we are just beginning to understand the benefits of eating fruits and vegetables.

POINTS TO REMEMBER

- Once a whole grain is refined, it no longer contains all the fiber and phytochemicals it used to have, and it no longer provides your body with the same level of disease prevention.

- It's okay to eat some refined flour and starches, but whole grains should make up most of the breads and cereals you eat every day.

- The fiber and phytochemicals found in whole foods appear to be able to reduce the risk of many chronic diseases.

- At least half of the breads and cereals you eat every day should be whole grain. The saying "Three are key" will also remind you to eat three servings of whole grains every day.

VEGETABLES ▶

FRUITS ▶

PLANTS ▶

VITAMINS ▶

PHYTOCHEMICALS ▶

OXYGEN ▶

FREE RADICALS ▶

ANTIOXIDANTS ▶

SUPPLEMENTS ▶

ONE-A-DAY VITAMINS ▶

/6

Thinking about Fruits and Vegetables in a Very Different Way

One has to question the wisdom of trying to improve what we don't understand.
—Unknown

YOU HAVE TO ADMIT THAT STUDIES that have looked at the health benefits of whole grains are impressive. It is hard to argue against eating more whole grains. But as good as these data are, the data supporting the benefits of consuming fruits and vegetables are even more convincing. You most likely already know about of the importance of getting vitamins and minerals from food—they are required for good nutrition. But as I mentioned earlier, plants have evolved and adapted to their environments, and in the process they've gained the ability to protect themselves from a variety of attacks by producing a variety of phytochemicals, specialized plant chemicals that are not found in animals or in meat or dairy products. Phytochemicals don't give you the energy, vitamins, or minerals you need for basic metabolism; phytochemicals play a different role. They are protectors of good health in that they defend against attackers that can damage and even kill you, plants, and other animals.

In 1982 the National Academy of Sciences reviewed all the existing research on fruits and vegetables and concluded that there appears to be a substantial health benefit associated with eating fruits and vegetables.[1] This marked the beginning of a wave of nutrition research on the importance of fruits and vegetables, and phytochemicals are currently the focus of most of that work.

Researchers have known for quite sometime that phytochemicals somehow provide protection for plants, but little was known about how plants could provide protection for humans. Large cohort studies of diet and disease have recently been completed and have consistently shown that diets that include ample fruits and vegetables are associated with dramatically lower rates of cancers, heart disease, stroke, and diabetes. Something in fruits and vegetables provided protection against disease, and phytochemicals appear to be the most likely candidates.

The amount of information about phytochemicals is impressive, but it will take many decades before we fully understand what they are, how they are produced, and how they work individually or together to ward off disease. At the present time, researchers have evaluated thousands of foods and have identified a little more than 5,000 different phytochemicals, but testing has shown that the total number of phytochemicals is likely to be far greater than 5,000, with most yet to be identified.[2]

One serving of vegetables may contain more than 100 different phytochemicals.

The number and type of phytochemicals in fruits, vegetables, and whole grains varies considerably from fruit to fruit, from vegetable to vegetable, and from whole grain to whole grain. One serving of vegetables may contain more than 100 different phytochemicals. Extensive studies have been done on onions, herbs, tomatoes, apples, broccoli, garlic, grapes, citrus fruit, and most other common fruits, vegetables, and whole grains, and research is currently ongoing to determine which foods have the most phytochemicals. But this should not convince someone to focus on any one food that is known to have a lot of phytochemicals because different phytochemicals are found in different foods,[3-5] and by focusing on one food, a person would likely fail to eat other valuable phytochemicals.

The identification of the different phytochemicals is occurring at a rapid pace, which means they don't always have a good naming system. Here is a list of some of the phytochemicals that have been identified:

phytoestrogens	alkaloids	indoles
isoprene	tannins	thiols
beta-carotene	saponins	silymarin
lycopene	terpenes	gingerols
lutein	phthalides	glycyrrhizin
zeaxanthin	allyl sulfides	flavinoids (3,000 types)
organosulfurs	glucosinolates	

And there are thousands more; the list goes on and on. The names alone are enough to make your head spin. If you are like me, you are glad that other people have devoted their life's work to studying things most people can't even pronounce.

Phytochemicals provide the color in the foods we eat. Think of all the colorful fruits and vegetables that are available. The bright yellow of a pepper or the orange of a carrot or a peach is caused by phytochemicals. Birds eat fruits, vegetables, and nuts and are able to use the phytochemicals to make their own color. A brightly colored parrot gets its color from the foods it eats. It has the right genetic blueprint to store phytochemicals in its feathers. Someone once asked me if they could get phytochemicals from eating the feathers of colorful birds. While they do contain lots of phytochemicals, once the phytochemicals have been used to provide color in a feather, human digestion cannot break them down. Besides, I think I'd be a little wary of anyone who liked the taste of feathers. Eating the meat won't do any good either because there are no phytochemicals in meat.

Phytochemicals are amazing. They come in different sizes—some are large, some are small. Some are positively charged while others are negatively charged. Some can be dissolved in water and others cannot. Some of them kill bacteria, viruses, or fungi. Some reduce inflammation just like over-the-counter anti-inflammatory drugs such as aspirin. Certain phytochemicals ward off insects.[6,7] These different characteristics give phytochemicals properties that are specific to certain disease-fighting processes. Perhaps the biggest benefit we get from consuming foods with phytochemicals, however, is their ability to stop oxidation. *Oxidation* is the fancy term to describe the changes oxygen can cause to other atoms, cells, and molecules.

Life with Oxygen: It's a Love-Hate Relationship

To convert the food we eat into usable energy for muscles and other organs, we need oxygen; without it we will die. But there is a darker, sinister side to oxygen. An oxygen atom has electrons spinning around it; all oxygen atoms are fond of their electrons and protect them. There is a strong bond that keeps oxygen atoms and their electrons together. During the normal processes of metabolism, an oxygen atom can lose an electron, and when this happens, the oxygen atom takes on a totally different personality.

INSIDE THE ALDANA HOME ►►► *When my wife and I had small children, we would pile into the car and take long road trips. One memorable trip took place when our youngest boy was nine months old. He had a strong affinity for his pacifier, just like an oxygen atom has for its electrons. After several hours of driving, boredom settled in, and an older brother reached over, grabbed the pacifier, and yanked it out of his mouth. Pop! You can probably guess what happened next. That beautiful little boy let out a scream that nearly cracked the front windshield and almost sent the car into a spin.*

In the excitement and confusion that followed, the pacifier got dropped somewhere in the back of the car and the screaming intensified. About this time, I was ready to join in with some screaming of my own. After a frantic search, the pacifier was no where to be found. Calmly, my brilliant wife opened the glove box and pulled out the "emergency" pacifier she had strategically hidden for just such an occasion. As soon as my son got it locked back into place between his trembling lips, the screaming stopped and everyone's heart rates returned to normal.

I recall watching three infants lined up in a row. The first did not have a pacifier, so he reached over and stole one from the little girl sitting next to him. The little girl became upset, then reached over to the next little girl and stole her pacifier, leaving her upset. I suppose they could play the pass-the-pacifier-along game so long as there was one to be stolen. This is exactly what happens at the atomic level. Once an oxygen atom loses an electron, the game of steal-an-electron-from-a-neighbor begins.

When an oxygen atom loses an electron, it travels around the body looking for any atom or molecule from which it can take an electron. However, the molecule or atom that made the "forced" donation is now lacking the right number of electrons and, like the infant whose pacifier was stolen, it prowls around for a replacement. This is the dark side of oxygen and of free radicals—the stealing of electrons starts a rash of thefts that can ultimately end in cell death or damage.

If an electron is taken from a protein that forms part of the structure of a cell wall, the cell will most likely die. If the electron is taken from a

We can't escape death, taxes, and oxidation.

You are more familiar with the process of oxidation than you think. When you cut an apple, it turns brown within minutes. Bananas that sit on the counter for a few days turn brown. Both of these are the result of oxidation. Rust that occurs on steel that has gotten wet or moist is also the result of oxidation.

vitamin, that vitamin can no longer perform its normal function. If an electron is taken from fat in the blood, it causes the fat to cling to artery walls; this is the first step in the process that leads to cardiovascular disease. If an electron is taken from a DNA strand within the nucleus of a cell, a mutation and, ultimately, cancer could occur. *It is estimated that the DNA material in every cell of the body is attacked by 10,000 free radicals every single day.*[8] Free radicals are also thought to be one of the causes of aging[9,10] and are a leading candidate in the search for the cause of Alzheimer's disease.[11-13]

If these free radicals are so bad, where do they all come from? Part of the answer makes perfectly good sense and part of it is a bit hard to take given the current state of our understanding of free radicals. Free radicals are produced by our own bodies during normal metabolism. We produce them every second of every day. The process of creating usable energy within muscles is another primary source of free radicals. That's right, you read this correctly: muscle activity needed for any physical activity produces free radicals. Since people who exercise have less cancer—not more—than those who are sedentary, it is obvious we don't completely understand what is going on yet.

Free radicals also come from the sun as ultraviolet light reaches our skin. They are produced by automobile exhaust, industrial chemicals, and other forms of air pollution. They are produced from radiation (including x-rays). They are found in burned foods, especially meat burned on an open flame. Perhaps most importantly, they are found in tobacco smoke. One puff of tobacco smoke has 100,000,000,000,000,000 (100 million billion) free radicals per puff.[14] This explains why smokers have such high rates of cardiovascular disease and cancer. This data also explains why secondhand smoke has been identified as a direct cause of cancer and asthma. In fact, if all smokers in the United States today quit smoking, there would be a 30% reduction in all cancers.[15] On more than one occasion I have presented this information and had smokers come up to me afterwards and say, "That's it, I'm done. I'm never going to smoke another cigarette as long as I live." I hope they were successful.

With this information about free radicals, it is tempting to start blaming free radicals for everything: depression, bipolar disorder, the common cold, rashes, and even cavities—all of these have been thrown onto the free radical bandwagon. While it is possible that many common disorders may have some association with free radicals, it is important to stick to known and accepted research.

How can phytochemicals help combat the impact of free radicals?

Some phytochemicals have the ability to donate an electron without being harmed by the process. It is as if they have an extra electron just waiting to be used during an emergency. These phytochemicals are called antioxidants because they can safely neutralize free radicals (oxidants). Vitamins B, C, D, E, and K also have antioxidant properties in addition to their important roles in good nutrition.

There is an even greater appeal in suggesting that phytochemicals are able to prevent a whole slew of common ailments. Many have gone to extremes to pronounce the lifesaving benefits of phytochemicals even though there is little data to support these claims. The research completed to date paints a very different picture than the one the public sees regarding the benefits of fruits and vegetables. This is almost exclusively due to the aggressive marketing and unregulated nature of supplement makers.

How Fruits and Vegetables Impact Your Life

Most scientists believe the benefits of eating fruits and vegetables come from their phytochemical and fiber content, but it is entirely possible that something else in them is responsible for protecting health. Regardless of the reason, people who regularly consume fruits and vegetables in addition to whole grains and nuts will have better health than those who do not; the data proves it.

Of all the people who die each year, one out of every four deaths is caused by cancer, and a poor diet, tobacco use, and lack of physical activity are responsible for 40–70% of all cancer deaths.[16,17] Let's put this into perspective. In 2001, 553,768 Americans died from cancer.[18] Of these deaths, as many as 387,637 (70% of all cancer deaths) could have been prevented or significantly delayed by a healthy diet, a tobacco-free lifestyle, and regular exercise. That's more than the total population of Miami, Florida, dying every single year.[19]

Diet seems to be the most important factor in predicting who might get cancer. In 1996, a review of every study ever conducted on cancer and nutrition evaluated the relationship between diet and cancer.[20] This review covered 206 studies that involved humans and 22 that involved animals. When the results of these studies are summarized, they provide evidence that consumption of fruits and vegetables can help protect against cancers of the stomach, esophagus, lung, oral cavity, pharynx, endometrium, pancreas, and colon.

When the people who consumed the most fruits and vegetables were compared to those who ate the least, they had half the cancer risk. The studies showed that fruits and vegetables stopped cancers at almost every stage of cancer growth, and the primary protective action is believed to be from phytochemicals. Another review of this research concluded that if Americans would consume five servings of fruits and/or vegetables each day, the prevalence of cancer could be cut in half.[21]

• •

SCIENCE MADE SIMPLE ►►► *The way this works is simple. Let's say you decide to eat an apple for lunch. From what we know right now, an apple contains over 100 different phytochemicals that enter your body after the apple is digested. Some of the phytochemicals are also antioxidants that are ready and willing to donate an extra electron to any free radical on the prowl for an electron it can claim as its own. (Remember, free radicals are not at all happy until they have the right number of electrons. If enough free radicals are neutralized, there are not as many hanging about looking to wreak havoc on some innocent DNA strand that is just minding its own business.) The apple you have eaten has eliminated a large number of free radicals and has helped reduce your cancer risk.*

• •

Now suppose that instead of eating an apple for lunch, you decide to eat a bowl of Apple Jacks cereal. This bowl of cereal contains only a tiny fraction of the phytochemicals found in the whole apple. Apple Jacks cereal does not cause cancer, but it also doesn't help prevent cancer like the whole apple does.

Dr. Rui Liu and his colleagues at Cornell University conducted some interesting studies on apples.[22] They isolated cancer cells and kept them in an environment that encouraged their growth. They then made three concentrated juices from just the skin of apples, just apple pulp, and skin and pulp combined. Each of these three juices was poured onto the growing cancer cells, and the researchers measured how fast the cells continued to grow. The cells with the juice from skins almost stopped dividing, the cells with the pulp juice kept on growing with no noticeable change, and the cells that got the pulp mixed with the skin (whole apple) slowed a moderate amount. So what does this mean? Did your mother ever tell you that you should eat the skin of your apple or baked potato? This study suggests that she was right after all. Chalk one up for moms!

This same study was conducted with grapes and the results were essentially the same. If you are going to eat fruit that has skin, eat the whole thing; the healthy phytochemicals appear to be concentrated in the skin.[23] Apples also have Vitamin C, which is an antioxidant, but when researchers evaluated all the antioxidant capacity of an apple, they found that less than one half of one percent of an apple's ability to fight free radicals comes from Vitamin C; the rest comes from the hundreds of other phytochemicals in the apple.[24]

People who regularly consume fruits, vegetables, whole grains, and nuts will have better health than those who do not; the data proves it.

There must be some truth to the saying, "An apple a day keeps the doctor away." Eating foods as close as possible to their natural form is the best way to protect against many of the most common forms of cancer. If you think about it, having phytochemicals concentrated in the skin makes sense. Any bacteria, virus, or other plant threat has to first penetrate the skin before the plant can be harmed. The skin on simple fruits and vegetables is far more complex than we might think.

It appears that fruits and vegetables are able to provide some protection against cardiovascular disease. If you compare the new cases of cardiovascular disease among people who eat 10 servings or more per day of fruits and vegetables with the cases among those who eat less than 2 servings, you find that those who eat a lot of fruits and vegetables have 20–30% lower risk.[25-27] Findings on strokes showed that for every serving of fruits or vegetables eaten per day, women get a 3% reduction in stroke risk and men get a 5% reduction in stroke risk.[28]

Even high blood pressure has been successfully lowered with a diet rich in fruits and vegetables, suggesting that if you have high blood pressure, the first thing to do is to starting eating more fruits and vegetables. If blood pressure does not come down to acceptable levels, work with your physician to try a blood pressure-lowering medication.[29]

Suppose you eat another apple. The phytochemicals that enter your body circulate around turning free radicals into pacifists. Some of those free radicals hoped to steal an electron from a molecule of LDL (bad cholesterol). Since the bad cholesterol molecule never gets altered, it never interacts with other molecules found in the walls of arteries, and the process of artery disease never starts.[30] Some free radicals like to make blood cells stick together, which makes blood flow more difficult, but that apple helped stop those guys, too.

While phytochemicals continue to circulate in your body, some of them eventually make it to your eyeballs. Over time and with exposure to light, the proteins that make up the lens of the eye can be damaged and the lens becomes cloudy. This is called a cataract. Some of the most recent research suggests that phytochemicals can dramatically delay the development of cataracts long enough for people to actually pass away before their cataracts worsen to the point that they need cataract surgery.[31]

As mentioned earlier, the tendency to want to blame free radicals for all that ails us and to promote phytochemicals as the solution to the world's problems is not a good idea. Research into phytochemicals is in its infancy, and it will take decades before we understand what is going on. Having said this, you should know that a few studies have been completed that suggest the possibility that fruits and vegetables may have other benefits. Some research has hinted that fruits and vegetables may slow or even prevent the cognitive and physical declines that are associated with aging,[32-34] degeneration of the retina,[35,36] diabetes,[37,38] and obesity.[39] Some of these health conditions may even turn out to be prevented by phytochemicals, but right now there is not enough good science to prove any of them.

Think of all the free radicals in your body as filling one half of a scale. The other side of the scale contains all the antioxidants and phytochemicals you consume in your diet. If you have a good diet, the scales stay balanced—you eat enough good foods to counter the free radicals being produced. If you fail to have a good diet, the free radicals side gets heavier and

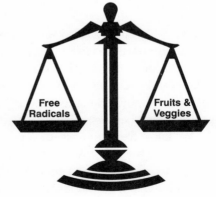

Free Radicals

Fruits & Veggies

the balance tips in favor of the free radicals. When this happens, your health leans toward the disease side of life. To keep the scales balanced, you have to eat whole foods.

Reality Check

It is one thing to talk about testing phytochemicals in laboratories. It is an entirely different thing to see if eating a healthy diet can prevent cancers in real people. In July 2004, researchers published data on a cohort study that included 30,000 women.[40] These women were followed for four years to see if those who ate a healthy diet had less cancer. Sure enough, in just four years, a healthy diet was related to a 22% reduction in new cancers and a significant reduction in cancer deaths. When smoking was also eliminated, new cancers were reduced by 30% and cancer deaths were reduced by 30%. These very recent results show that a healthy diet can have a substantial impact on reducing new cancers and cancer deaths. It appears that what scientists are finding in the laboratory appears to be true in the real world: a healthy diet can prevent cancers.

Just How Many Fruits and Vegetables Should You Eat?

Just because a little of something is good, it is not always true that a lot of something is better—unless you are talking about fruits and vegetables. The National Cancer Institute recommends that every American get five servings of fruits and/or vegetables per day as a minimum, and even more is better. I've heard Dr. Ken Cooper from the Cooper Aerobics Center in Dallas, Texas, say, "Eating five will keep you alive, but nine is divine." That's quite a statement from America's top exercise guru.

National surveys show that 78% of Americans don't even eat five servings per day, much less experience the divine; the average American eats 2.7 servings of fruits and/or vegetables each day. With all the fruits and vegetables that are available fresh, frozen, or even canned, can you guess what the two most commonly consumed fruits and/or vegetables are? French fries and ketchup. (Ketchup counts because it is made from tomatoes.) That means that a good portion of the servings of fruits and vegetables Americans eat each day are in the form of french fries and ketchup. This is a great example of the enormous gap that exists between what we know and what we actually do.

We know fruits and vegetables are good for us, but we just can't seem to overcome the pressure to eat otherwise. Given the poor diet of most Americans, I believe that a goal to eat the minimum—five servings per day—is realistic. That means if you eat five servings of fruits or five servings of vegetables or five servings of a combination of fruits and vegetables, you will start to enjoy all the benefits we've discussed. If you will eat more than that, you will experience even greater disease protection and health promotion. (Don't forget to read chapter 12. It will give you great ideas to successfully make fruits and vegetables part of your daily diet.)

If getting Americans to eat fruits and vegetables is so hard, why can't all those brilliant scientists find a way to isolate those healthy antioxidants and phytochemicals, put them in a pill, and give the pills to the public? That's a great question.

The Public Wants a Pill

Conflict abounds at the point where scientific evidence and American capitalism cross. Business owners want to make money, scientists want to discover truth, and the rest of us sit in the bleachers and try to sort fact from fiction, truth from aggressive marketing, and scientific enthusiasm from rampant greed. I decided to write this book to empower wise consumers. I'm giving you the science and hoping you will make wise choices regarding your body and your health.

In 2000, the vitamin and supplement industry generated $16.8 billion in retail sales. This largely unregulated industry has grown every single year since data was recorded. The marketing of their products is intense, but the current state of the science behind their products is not nearly as clear as they might have you believe. A myriad of studies have been completed that have evaluated the effects of supplements on a variety of health issues. There is so much research in this area that many books have been written on this topic alone. To answer the question of whether or not the perfect pill can be created, let's look at one small segment of this research.

In chapter 2 you learned about the difficult nature of doing research. The figure on page 26 shows the results of all the studies that have looked at physical activity and breast cancer. You will recall that most of the studies showed that physical activity appeared to protect against breast cancer, but there were a few studies that failed to find this result. Well, in much the same way, there have been over 72 different studies that have looked at the relationship between tomatoes, tomato-based foods, and cancer.[41] Among other things, tomatoes contain lycopene, a phytochemical and antioxidant. Contrary to what you may have heard, lycopene and the other phytochemicals found in tomatoes are actually more available if the tomatoes have been processed. Yes, you read it right—boiling the heck out of tomatoes actually makes them better for you, not worse.[40] (But I still love my fresh tomatoes.)

Of the 72 studies on tomatoes, 57 found that the more tomatoes you eat, the lower your cancer risk. The other 15 studies showed that tomato consumption made no difference, and not a single study showed that eating tomatoes increased cancer risk.

Here is where the research is clear, but the supplement industry gets a little ahead of itself. Lycopene is only one of hundreds of phytochemicals found in tomatoes, and there is no evidence that the lycopene alone is directly responsible for the protection afforded from tomatoes.[41] It is possible that lycopene by itself is responsible for the reduction in cancer risk, but that is doubtful. More realistically, the cancer protection benefits of lycopene can be gained only if lycopene works in conjunction with all the other components of tomatoes. When the best researchers in the world clearly warn that our understanding of lycopene is in its infancy and that use of supplements containing purified lycopene is extremely premature and possibly dangerous, the public should listen and be cautious.

Americans are easy prey for supplement makers, but don't get suckered in.

Unfortunately, in their search for greater corporate profits, supplement makers don't care much about expert opinions. Because they have to comply with very few FDA regulations, they grab hold of the lycopene research and practically stumble over themselves to get lycopene purified, encapsulated, and on the shelves for the public to use. Worst of all, they are so aggressive in their advertising and marketing that the unsuspecting public buys the marketing stories hook, line, and sinker. While scientists are saying, "Whoa, we don't know what is going on yet," supplement makers flood the airways with the "latest and greatest secret to good health."

If you watch television commercials, you will see advertisements promoting beta-carotene, lycopene, selenium, and other phytochemicals. As the evidence of the health benefits of phytochemicals continues to grow, Americans are easy prey for supplement makers,[42] but don't get suckered in. The wisest thing to do is to eat whole grains and at least five servings of fruits and/or vegetables every day.

Why a Fruit-and-Veggie Pill Is a Bad Idea

There are thousands of phytochemicals in the plant foods we eat and only a portion of these have been identified. Lycopene is only one of the possibly hundreds of phytochemicals found in tomatoes; we have yet to identify all the components of even a simple tomato. A supplement that includes just lycopene has missed not only the other phytochemicals found in tomatoes that we know about, but also the ones we don't know about. Unless you eat whole foods, all the supplementation in the world will still leave you without the vast majority of the health-promoting parts of plant foods. You run the risk of not consuming something your body needs to stay healthy.

Experts also agree that it appears that phytochemicals need to work with other phytochemicals to be effective. They seem to need and to complement each other, but the complex interactions that exist between these compounds are presently unknown. Furthermore, it is impossible to isolate one of thousands of compounds found in a food and expect that compound to work independent of all the other phytochemicals that were originally part of the same whole food.

Modern science has been attempting to study the effects of individual phytochemicals. Some of the findings look promising—that's why the supplement industry has been so aggressive—but there is a large and growing amount of research that shows that phytochemical supplementation has a darker, dangerous side. You won't see commercials about these studies, and I promise you won't be reading about them on the back of your cereal box. I suspect you will find this information hard to believe because we have all been exposed to the media's continual praise for antioxidants. When doing research, things don't always go the way you expect them to.

In an extremely large randomized study, 18,000 current and former smokers were given either a placebo or a supplement of beta-carotene and Vitamin A. The study was supposed to last for six years, but it was terminated after just four years. What the researchers found was extremely disappointing for supplement manufacturers and pharmaceutical companies, both of whom had hoped to cash in on a "magic bullet of health." The participants who took the beta-carotene supplement were 28% more likely to get lung cancer, 46% more likely to die of lung cancer, and 26% more likely to die of cardiovascular disease. That's right, instead of improving health, the supplement was directly responsible for more cancer and premature death.[43]

The public perceives that Vitamin C is most likely a harmless supplement, but the blood of 30 study volunteers suggests a different picture. After taking 500 mg of Vitamin C every day for three weeks, cellular DNA strands of those who took Vitamin C showed more damage than cellular

DNA strands from the group who didn't take Vitamin C. The group taking Vitamin C was actually disrupting the DNA in their white blood cells![44] Other studies of Vitamin C reported that the supplements also had no effect on cancer or heart disease.

Long-term supplementation of beta-carotene had no effect on preventing other cancers and cardiovascular disease[45] and supplementation with Vitamin E revealed that the supplement did nothing to prevent cancer, heart disease, or stroke.[46,47] These few studies must be considered with other studies that showed possible health benefits of some antioxidants. Until more is known, the prudent thing to do is to eat whole foods.

What about a One-a-Day Vitamin?

The risks and benefits of taking a one-a-day vitamin have also been studied extensively, and the best researchers in the world are split in their opinions. One group, the U.S. Preventive Services Task Force, has concluded, "There is insufficient scientific evidence to recommend vitamin supplements as a way to prevent cancer or heart disease. Vitamin supplements may be necessary for individuals whose diets don't provide the recommended amounts of specific vitamins and especially important for pregnant and nursing women and people with specific illnesses. However, the benefits of vitamin supplements for the general population remain uncertain."[48]

One year earlier, a prominent physician writing in one of the nation's top medical journals suggested, "Most people do not consume an optimal amount of all vitamins by diet alone and should take a multi-vitamin."[49] This opinion is shared by many other prominent nutritionists. My advice is to eat a balanced, whole-foods diet. If for some reason you absolutely don't want the health benefits of good food and don't have a good diet, a multi-vitamin probably won't hurt you.

POINTS TO REMEMBER

- Our understanding of the functions of phytochemicals and free radicals is very limited.

- Everyday the DNA in our cells gets attacked 10,000 times by free radicals. Phytochemicals can neutralize free radicals and help prevent cancer.

- Eating at least five or more servings of fruits and/or vegetables every day provides significant protection against many cancers and other diseases; even more than five servings per day is better.

- Whole foods are incredibly complex. Scientists are just beginning to figure out how our bodies use everything that is in the food we eat.

- Consuming individual phytochemicals in supplements is not recommended; the only way to get the best possible health is to eat fruits and vegetables.

7

Swapping Bad Fats for Good Health

The need for change bulldozed a road down the center of my mind.
—Maya Angelou (1928–)

INSIDE THE ALDANA HOME ►►► *When I was a child growing up in Idaho, I ate a bowl of ice cream every day after dinner. My parents would buy it in large, three-gallon containers. Because the containers were so big and handy, my mother would save them. The lids made great frisbees and the containers made great drums. On most mornings I ate eggs, bacon, and heavily buttered toast and drank a big glass of whole milk straight from the dairy down the street. Neither I nor my parents ever thought there was anything wrong with the way we were eating. After all, this was the same way my grandparents ate; it was the way my friends ate; it was part of my cultural and family heritage. That was life in Idaho.*

Other cultures in the United States are not without their high-fat foods. Southerners are known for their hospitality and food that often includes fried foods, barbecue, biscuits and gravy, and lots of meat. Texas is known for its superb cattle industry, which believes plentiful grasses and proper animal care provide the finest steaks in the world.

One of the hardest parts about living a healthy lifestyle is trying to adjust our cultural and ethnic identities to what is known about good health. To most people that means asking, "What do I have to 'give up' in order to be healthy?" Well, there is no simple way to achieve good health. It takes some adjustment and change—and, yes, it might even require some drastic changes in the way we live.

For example, to have good health it is not a good idea to smoke. If you do smoke, you should quit—the sooner, the better—and you should never smoke again. You will also need to completely forsake your smoker's lifestyle. This might mean no longer going to locations where smoking might be a temptation, finding something else to do besides smoke, and maybe even throwing out all your ashtrays, matches, and unused cigarettes. This is a drastic solution to a very dangerous health issue, but it is the best way for the 23% of Americans who smoke to dramatically improve their health.

Humans don't have to smoke to live, but they do have to eat. Since we have to eat, all that is really needed for a healthier diet is to change the types of foods we eat. I still eat breakfast everyday, but I don't eat the foods I used to eat, and ice cream is only an occasional indulgence.

The Dietary Fat Hit List

Dietary fat has been on the nutrition hit list for about 20 years. Today we see the battle against fat everywhere we go. Jared, the spokesperson for Subway sandwiches, has been leading the way to healthy body weight by eating low-fat, healthy Subway sandwiches. He claims to have eaten low-fat Subway sandwiches every day and lost over 100 pounds as a result. Lay's offers potato chips that are baked rather than fried like traditional potato chips; Frito-Lay's sales of the chips has exploded. There is low-fat ice cream, low-fat chocolate, low-fat salad dressing—just about everything that used to be high in fat now has a low-fat version.

Research in the past had formed a picture of good health, and excessive dietary fat wasn't in the picture. Studies of the effects of diet on cancer in rodents had shown that different amounts of dietary fat could change the rate at which cancers could grow, and researchers could predict the total number of cancers these animals would get.[3] And saturated fat, the type of fat that comes from animals and is solid at room temperature, was shown to have strong ties to heart disease because it increased bad cholesterol.[4-6] It was also clear to health experts that the countries that consumed the most fat also had the highest rates of certain cancers and cardiovascular disease,[7] leading health authorities to start recommending that saturated fat be

Fake fats

Olean is a "fake fat," which is used in commercially produced foods. The digestive system thinks these fake fats are real fats and tries to digest them but cannot. So while they taste like fat to us, they pass through our digestive systems impervious to our bodies' attempts to digest them.[1] That these fake fats are so close to the real thing that our bodies are completely fooled is actually an amazing property. But even though fake fats may have some good properties, like taste, it appears they may not be healthy. Research on individuals who have been eating fake fats shows a reduction in the number of phyotochemicals in their bodies.[2] Vitamins and phytochemicals that are in the foods we eat aren't automatically absorbed into the bloodstream during digestion. To get through the intestinal wall, they have to bind with a fat, which acts like an escort. Together, they cross the intestinal wall and enter the bloodstream. Without fat in your diet, vitamins and phytochemicals can't get into your blood and help keep you healthy. When phytochemicals and vitamins attach to fake fats, they think they are getting a ride through the intestinal wall and into the blood, but in reality the only ride they are getting is a one-way trip on the porcelain express. And because they are not absorbed by your body, you don't get any benefit. Though the FDA currently allows fake fats to be used in processed foods, they have yet to allow fast food manufacturers to use them to fry foods. Until the entire effects of these designer foods are better understood, the prudent thing to do would be to avoid them.

limited. Despite intense efforts to make the best recommendations, dietary fat was blackballed and placed on the nutrition hit list with other publicly recognized health concerns, and the message that evolved as a result is that all fats are bad.

This message has been the call to action for many food manufacturers, health programs, and popular diet and health programs, and there has been some success. The Dean Ornish Heart Disease Reversing Program requires program participants to eat a plant-based diet and to limit dietary fat to no more than 10% of all calories.[8] That is extremely low considering the average American consumes about 34% of total calories from fat. Most Ornish Program participants start the program with advanced stages of cardiovascular disease and if they can exercise, maintain the diet, and practice stress management, there is evidence that they can actually unblock plugged arteries and dramatically improve heart health. Other programs that appear to have had success with the "all fats are bad" message are the Pritikin Program and the Coronary Heart Improvement Program (CHIP).[9,10]

Low-fat diets also appear to be helpful for individuals who are trying to lose weight or maintain weight loss.[11] There are many individuals who have lost significant amounts of body fat and maintained the weight loss for several years. 3,000 of these long-term weight loss success stories are documented as part of a national weight loss database called the National Weight Control Registry. When asked how they were successful at keeping the weight off, registry members identified two key behaviors: regular physical activity and a low-fat diet. Low-fat diets appear to have some effect on long-term weight loss and cardiovascular disease, but if you seriously consider the more recent nutrition evidence, it is obvious that the "all fats are bad" message needs to be updated.

Fat Increases While Fat Decreases

Under the all-fats-are-bad diet, fats are cut from the diet and have to be replaced with either more protein or carbohydrates. The low-fat diets and health programs mentioned previously aim to replace the fat calories with additional calories from whole grains, fruits, and vegetables. This is a great trade-off. Perhaps that is why these programs have been able to demonstrate improved health and weight loss. However, when the public cuts dietary fat, the fat is most likely replaced with simple carbohydrates or sugars, not health-promoting whole foods.

Since 1965, there has been a decline in the percent of total calories that come from fat. Today, men and women consume approximately 32% of their calories from fat, whereas 40 years ago dietary fat accounted for 45% of all the calories eaten.[12,13] During this same time period, the percent of Americans who are obese or overweight has been increasing. The decrease in dietary fat and the increase in weight are shown in Figure 7.1. You would think that if people are eating less fat, they would weigh less, but obviously this is not the case when we look at the entire U.S. population.

Physical activity during this time has been relatively unchanged, with only 25% of Americans getting the recommended amount of physical activity. Since 1971, the total number of calories being eaten every day per person has increased by about 168 calories for men and about 335 for women.[13] That means men are eating an amount equivalent to three apples more and the women are eating the equivalent of five apples more each day than they did in 1971. Most of these increased calories are believed to come

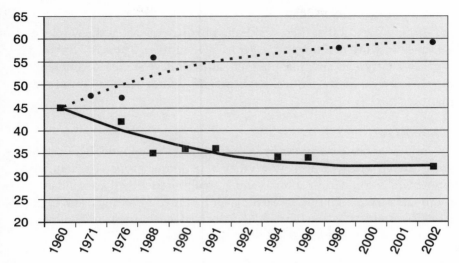

Figure 7.1 Increases in body weight and decreases in dietary fat in the United States. The dashed line indicates the trend in the percent of adults who are overweight or obese; the solid line indicates the trend in the percentage of calories from fat over the same period.[12-14]

from eating salty snacks, soft drinks, pizza, more foods away from home, and increased portion sizes.[15,16]

Let's try to make some sense of this data. The nation's physical activity has stayed the same, dietary fat has come down, daily calories consumed have increased, and as a nation, we are fatter now than at any other point in history. It is tempting to look at this graph and conclude that the reductions we've experienced in dietary fat are somehow causing the dramatic increases in weight being experienced by Americans. Unfortunately, we don't know if this is the case because there are many other possible explanations for this apparent link.

For example, during this same time frame, food has become more affordable, with even the poorest in our society consuming too many calories. Food has also become more convenient, with the number of fast food restaurants continuing to grow, and the size of food servings has increased dramatically. This period also corresponds to the era of the "free refill."

The number of calories consumed per person has also increased over this same time period, suggesting that the fat that has been reduced in our diets is being replaced with carbohydrates and protein. This substitution does not appear to be an equal trade of calories—it is more of a small reduction in fat calories for a large increase in other calories.

Sorting Out Fats from Fiction

You will recall that there are many phytochemicals in the whole foods we eat—so many that most have yet to be identified. The basic unit of fat is called a fatty acid and, like phytochemicals, there are many different types. Based on their chemical structure, most fatty acids fall into four main categories.

Saturated Fats

Saturated fats have all the hydrogen atoms they can hold. Because they are saturated with hydrogen atoms they have unique properties. Saturated fats generally come from animals and animal products and are solid at room temperature. Butter, shortening, fat trimmed from meat, and high-fat dairy products have saturated fat. Saturated fats raise blood cholesterol, which increases the risk of heart disease and stroke.

Monounsaturated Fats

These fats are really oils. They are liquid at room temperature but get more solid when they are stored in the refrigerator. Chemists call the most common monounsaturated fat cis-9-octadecenoic acid. Physiologists call it oleic acid. Olive oil is mostly monounsaturated fat. Olive oil can be mixed with vinegar to make an oil-and-vinegar salad dressing. This dressing is liquid at room temperature, but when it's stored in the refrigerator, it starts to solidify and becomes cloudy. When substituted for saturated fat in a person's diet, monounsaturated fats appear to lower blood cholesterol, which means they are actually good for you.

Polyunsaturated Fats

Unless you get these fats from your diet, your body cannot produce them on its own. These fats differ chemically from monounsaturated fats. They are liquid both at room temperature and when kept in the refrigerator. For some reason, polyunsaturated fats actually help lower total blood cholesterol and are heart healthy. One of the most commonly talked about polyunsaturated fats is 4,7,10,13,16,19-docosahexaenoic acid or DHA, a nasty name for what the public calls fish oil. Polyunsaturated fats are also very common in seeds, plant oils, and whole grains.

Trans Fats

These fats are a little different from the ones above. They are polyunsaturated fats that have been altered in a process called hydrogenation. In this process, healthy vegetable oils are heated to about 400 degrees and hydrogen gas and a metal catalyst are added. This makes the unsaturated vegetable oil accept additional hydrogen atoms, and, presto, what used to be an unsaturated fat is now a saturated fat with special properties. It can be used over and over again to fry food without going rancid, and it has a very long shelf life. Trans fats are found in processed cookies, cakes, fried foods, and bakery goods. Trans fats increase bad cholesterol more than unsaturated fats.

Foods containing the four types of fats			
Saturated fat	Monounsaturated fat	Polyunsaturated fat	Trans fat
cheese	olive oil	safflower oil	margarine
whole milk	canola oil	corn oil	vegetable shortening
dark chocolate	peanut butter	sunflower oil	any deep-fried foods
butter	almonds	soybean oil	french fries
ice cream	nuts	corn	most bakery goods
fatty meats	avocados	fish	anything made
coconut milk	sesame seeds	walnuts	with shortening
lard	pumpkin seeds		or partially
			hydrogenated
			vegetable oil

INSIDE THE ALDANA HOME ▶▶▶ *Many years ago I was working at Oklahoma State University. My family and I loved living in Oklahoma because everyone was always so nice and friendly. My oldest son had tasted beef spare ribs during dinner at a friend's home and wondered if our family could go to dinner and have ribs. After much pleading, I gave in and took the family to one of the famous barbecue rib restaurants that are so popular in the Midwest. My son ordered a rack of barbecued beef ribs. As he was enjoying his ribs, the juices from the meat and barbecue sauce ran down his arm and made a small pool on the table. He really liked the ribs. As we finished dinner and had some time to visit, my son noticed that the small pool of juice that had dripped down his arm and onto the table had hardened. It looked like wax from a candle; in fact, he thought it was wax.*

This was one of those moments when I was able to explain the difference between saturated fat and unsaturated fat. At cooking temperature, the fat from the ribs was liquid and could run like water, but after it cooled to room temperature, it hardened. If the same pool of juice had been placed in a refrigerator it would have hardened even more.

Think about the foods you eat during the day. Which ones contain fat and how can you tell? Well, deep-fried foods, bakery goods, butter, high-fat dairy products (like cheese and ice cream), and any food that leaves a shine on your fingers after you eat it are high-fat foods. Salad dressings, fatty meats (like bacon and steaks), peanut butter, and french fries are also high in fat. However, just because a food is high in fat doesn't mean it should be avoided. There are good fats and there are bad fats. The trick is to eat a diet that reduces one and increases the other.

Why You Should Care about Good Fats and Bad Fats

I know this next section may be difficult to believe, but try to forget all the hard work and time you have spent identifying and eliminating high-fat foods from your diet. Try at least to consider the evidence before you make a decision about what you should and should not eat. As we discussed earlier, there is some limited support for the all-fats-are-bad approach to good health. When all fats are treated equally, dietary fat appears to be related to several chronic diseases. But we have discovered that all fats are not the same. Each of the four main types of fat behaves differently.

In 1997, Dr. Frank Hu at Harvard published findings from the Nurses' Health Study that gave a great example of these differences.[17] After following the lifestyle choices of 80,000 women for 14 years, the relationship between dietary fat and coronary heart disease was studied. The diets of all these women were monitored and the amounts of total, saturated, trans, polyunsaturated, and monounsaturated fats were measured. These measures of dietary fat were then used to determine the risk of having heart disease. When the health information from women with high-fat diets was compared to the information from women with low-fat diets, there was no difference in the risk of coronary heart disease. But when the different types of fat were looked at independently, a very different picture emerged.

While polyunsaturated fats reduced heart disease risk by 38% and monounsaturated fats reduced the risk by 19%, both saturated and trans fats increased heart disease risk. Those who ate the most saturated fat had a 17% greater risk of heart disease compared to those who ate the least. Those who ate the most trans fats had a 93% increase in heart disease risk—almost 5.5 times greater than the risk associated with saturated fat. You can guess which of these fats are good and which are bad.

Taken individually, these four types of fat reveal a stark disparity in the way our bodies handle fats (see Figure 7.2). Good fats (polys and monos) tend to offset bad fats (saturated and trans). Past studies of the effect of

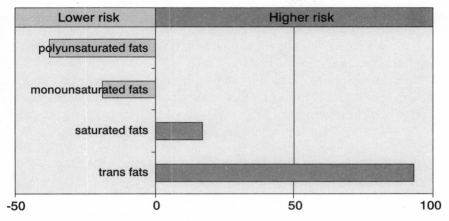

Figure 7.2 Good fats decrease and bad fats increase heart disease risk in women[17]

total fat didn't recognize that the benefits of the good fats cancelled out the harmful effects of the bad fats.

Good Fats

Polyunsaturated fats have been studied quite extensively and can be further classified into plant oils and fish oils. Plant oils come from corn, sunflower, canola, and other plant sources such as nuts. Peanut butter is a good source of polyunsaturated fat. Plant oils have shown some remarkable tendencies to protect our bodies from chronic diseases. A diet that includes nuts and peanut butter can reduce the risk of diabetes by 21%.[18,19] To get this much protection, you would have to eat only about a half a cup of nuts every week. That is not very much if you spread it out over seven days.

Individuals who increase the amount of polyunsaturated fat in their diets experience several changes in their metabolism. Bad cholesterol (LDL) goes down, good cholesterol (HDL) goes up, and total cholesterol can drop by as much as 6%.[20] These improvements in blood cholesterol translate into a 12–44% reduction in the risk of heart disease, stroke, and other vessel diseases.[21-24]

Other studies have looked at how polyunsaturated fats might affect overall health. A study of older adults showed that eating high amounts of polyunsaturated fats could reduce the risk of Alzheimer's disease. The same study showed that those who eat higher amounts of saturated fats and trans fats double their risk of getting Alzheimer's as they age.[25] At the present time, there is no clear data showing that polyunsaturated fats can prevent cancer, and a few studies have even suggested the possibility that polyunsaturated fats may be linked with prostate cancer.[26] Obviously, much more research is needed before this part of the fat puzzle is completely understood.

Think of monounsaturated fat as polyunsaturated fat's little brother. They both act in similar ways. Both increase good cholesterol, decrease bad cholesterol, and reduce the risk of cardiovascular diseases. They are both liquid at room temperature, and both can be found in plant oils. It is almost impossible to get one without the other. When you think of monounsaturated fats, think of olive oil, which is mostly monounsaturated fat.

In the 1960s, researchers looked at death and disease rates in different countries and discovered a group of people who, despite having poor medical care, had the longest life spans in the world. They also had some of the lowest rates of heart disease, cancers, diabetes, and obesity found anywhere. These healthy souls were the citizens of Crete, Greece, and Southern Italy, and they all shared a Mediterranean lifestyle.

The traditional diet in these areas consisted of an abundance of plant foods, including nuts, breads, pastas, beans, and fruits and vegetables. The diet also included some fish, poultry, dairy foods, meat, eggs, and wine and was low in sweets. Olive oil was the primary source of fat in this diet, which also had almost no trans fats and was low in saturated fats and high in monounsaturated fats. In the 1960s this was the traditional diet of the general population. Since that time, however, the diet has become increasingly Westernized so that today the traditional Mediterranean diet has become a hybrid diet in which fast foods and processed foods have become a substantial part of the regional diet.

Monounsaturated fats get most of their fame and attention from the health-promoting role they play in the traditional Mediterranean diet. They are believed to be responsible for much of the health benefits experienced in the region.[27] Parts of Italy, France, Portugal, Spain, Tunisia, Turkey, and Morocco also enjoy variations of this diet, but few are still completely true to their Mediterranean roots.

The Mediterranean diet appears to prevent chronic diseases in several ways. The good monounsaturated fats help keep blood cholesterol levels and the risk of heart and vessel disease low. An abundance of fruits, vegetables, and whole grains introduces a variety of antioxidants and phytochemicals into the body, which may also help prevent vessel disease, but the diet is also believed to prevent cancers, diabetes, obesity, and possibly Alzheimer's disease. Additionally, olive oil, fish oil, and other whole foods may decrease colon and breast cancer risk.

One way to really see if the Mediterranean diet is really that good would be to have people adopt the diet and track them across time, which is exactly what French researchers did.[28] They convinced 600 men and women who already had heart disease to try either a Mediterranean diet or a diet from the American Heart Association. The 4-year study was stopped after just 2.5 years because the effects of the diet were obvious and there was no need to continue. The group that started on the Mediterranean diet showed a 70% reduction in deaths from all causes—pretty good evidence that the diet is responsible for much of the good health in the Mediterranean region.

Learning from the Eskimos

Years ago, researchers working in the Arctic were surprised to learn that Eskimos rarely die of heart disease despite a diet extremely high in animal fat. It was believed at that time that animal fat was the same among animals and that if you ate a lot of animal fat, you were asking for heart disease; not so among the Eskimos. Since this early observation, much has been learned about the type of fat consumed by Eskimos. It is a type of polyunsaturated fat we refer to as fish oils. Unlike the juicy ribs my son liked so much, the oil from fish, especially cold-water fish like salmon and tuna, does not harden when it reaches room temperature; it is chemically different. The same types of fats are found in smaller amounts in seeds and walnuts and in soybean and canola oils.

These fats help keep the heart beating properly,[29,30] which might not seem like a big deal—unless you know that many of the heart disease deaths that occur each year are caused by a sudden change in the heart's normal beating. The beat suddenly becomes rapid and irregular, and the first sign that anything is wrong is sudden death. Most sudden cardiac deaths occur this way. We are not exactly sure why, but in humans and in animals, those who eat higher amounts of polyunsaturated fats maintain regular heart beats.

At the time this book was being written, 19 studies had been published that looked at the relationship between fish intake and coronary heart disease.[31] The participants in these studies were categorized as those who ate fish and those who ate little or no fish. Fish eaters had about 15% less risk of both heart disease and heart disease death; this is believed to be due to the healthy fish oils. These oils also help prevent blood from clotting, which reduces the chance of having a blocked artery, and they improve blood cholesterol.

Several studies that encouraged individuals to eat more of this healthy fat have been published. They all generally agree that sudden cardiac death can be prevented, but that it is unclear if heart attacks in general, cancers, or strokes are affected.[32,33] The added protection available from eating fish is why fish is included in the Healthy Eating Pyramid shown in chapter 5.

Bad Fats

Figure 7.2 shows the relationship between heart disease risk and the four types of fat. If you were to rank the fats from best to worst, your list would look like this: polys, monos, saturated, and trans, implying that each is only slightly worse than the next. In reality, the scientific evidence available today suggests that trans fats are far worse than the other three, at least as far as heart disease risk is concerned. Most of the research that has been completed in this area has focused on saturated fat, which has been identified as one of the two unhealthy fats that are part of our diets. Saturated fat has received this reputation because study after study has suggested that individuals who have diets high in saturated fat are also at greater risk for heart disease, stroke, diabetes, breast cancer, and maybe colon and prostate cancers.[34-41] Saturated fat has also been implicated as one of the causes of Alzheimer's disease[42] and appears possibly to be associated with schizophrenia.[43]

The biggest sources of saturated fats are animal products. Red meat and high-fat dairy products like whole milk, cheese, butter, and ice cream are leading sources of saturated fat. From the plant world, palm kernel oil, coconut oil, and coconut milk are also high in saturated fats. Saturated fat is found in other plant oils and plants as well, but in much smaller quantities.

To see how much saturated fat is really in your diet, you have to look at the labels on the foods you eat. We won't spend time learning how to read the labels here, but I highly recommend that you go to the FDA's Web site and use their well-designed guides to learn how to evaluate food labels. (You can find the site on the Web at www.cfsan.fda.gov/label.html.) Food labels tell you how many grams of saturated fat are in each serving of the food you are eating. The best guidelines to date suggest that you should not let saturated fats be more than 10% of all the calories you eat per day.

In general, women should eat no more than 20 grams of total fat per day and men should eat less than 25 grams. Look closely at labels and you quickly see how much saturated fat the food contains. If you have a food you are not sure about, you can most likely find the label on the Web at www.nutritiondata.com. You can even look up fast foods at this site.

It's time for a little quiz. Here is a label from a popular snack. Evaluate the label for saturated fat and decide if you want to eat it.

Nutrition Facts

Serving Size: 128g

Amount Per Serving	
Calories 520	Calories from Fat 189
	%DV*
Total Fat 21g	32%
Saturated Fat 11g	55%
Cholesterol 15mg	5%
Sodium 400mg	17%
Total Carbohydrate 79g	26%
Dietary Fiber 2g	8%
Sugars 29g	
Protein 3g	6%

Can you guess what it is? It's a Hostess fruit pie. One pie contains 11 grams of saturated fat. No, you won't die if you eat it. But if the rest of your diet during the day includes other foods with saturated fats, you will most likely consume too much saturated and trans fats. It's great to indulge in an occasional treat, but keep an eye on the labels; they tell you what you are really eating. Your health is determined by the overall quality of your diet, not by any one item you may eat.

Trans Fats

Research findings in the past few years have identified trans fats as a serious threat to good health. In fact, trans fats are quickly becoming public health enemy number one. Of all the calories Americans eat, just about 3% come from trans fats. Trans fats are manufactured, so they appear most often in processed foods. Of all the trans fats in our diets, half come from cakes, cookies, crackers, pies, and bread. The rest come from animal products, margarine, fried potatoes, potato chips, corn chips, high-fat popcorn, shortening, breakfast cereal, and candy.

Food producers use trans fats instead of healthier unsaturated fats because foods prepared with trans fats stay fresh longer and have a texture most people like. For example, margarine, which is mostly made from trans fats, is softer than real butter and easier to work with. Pie crusts, crackers, and croissants are flakier when made with trans fats, and it is cheaper to fry foods in trans fats because they last much longer than unsaturated frying oils.

If you compare a gram of saturated fats and a gram of trans fats, trans fats impose a risk of heart disease that is 10 times greater than the risk associated with saturated fats. Four very large cohort studies revealed approximately the same results.[17,44-46] The consumption of trans fats was positively associated with a 25% increase in heart disease risk.

From 1977 to 1995, the number of heart disease deaths in Denmark was cut by half, and during the exact same time, the entire population of Denmark cut its consumption of trans fats by 75%.[47] These two trends may be related. Nine different studies compared the effect of saturated fat and trans fats on both good and bad cholesterol.[48] Both decreased the good and increased the bad cholesterol, but the effect of the trans fats was 2.5 times worse than the effect of the saturated fats, suggesting that saturated fats are bad but trans fats are much worse.

Nuts: No longer dietary bad boys

One of the unfortunate side effects of the all-fats-are-bad message has been the demise of nuts in the American diet. As you've read, nuts are a high-fat food containing mostly good fats, some saturated fats, and no trans fats. In the last 10 years considerable research has shown that nuts might have been unfairly singled out, and they should be reintroduced into the American diet. Nuts and peanut butter have now been identified as having the ability to lower the risk of heart disease and diabetes.[50,51] Women who ate peanut butter five times a week or more had a 21% reduction in the risk of getting diabetes.[18] A diet that included walnuts caused the arteries of the participants to be more responsive to changes in blood pressure,[52] and a diet high in macadamia nuts improved blood cholesterol.[53]

When trying to help patients lower blood cholesterol, doctors are generally quick to prescribe a blood cholesterol-lowering medication. However, in a head-to-head study that compared patients on a healthy diet that included nuts with patients who were only on medication, there was no difference between the two groups. Both the patients on the healthy diet and the patients on the medication saw their blood cholesterol drop about 30%.[54] The group on the healthy diet also got the added benefits of whole grains, fruits, vegetables, and healthy fats.

There are two concerns often expressed with eating nuts. One is that they may cause allergies in some people, and the other is that they are calorie dense and might cause people to gain weight. Peanuts and nuts that grow on trees can cause allergic reactions in some people. It is estimated that possibly 1% of adults may have an allergic response.[55] If you are in this group, you may need to monitor your consumption of nuts.

Weight gain from eating a diet with nuts is so far unfounded.[56,57] In studies where participants were forced to eat diets high in nuts, none of the participants gained weight. Studies that gave people the option of eating a diet with nuts found that participants actually lost a little weight. Even though it appears no one is gaining weight from eating nuts, it still might be safe to substitute nuts for sugars or refined flour already in excess in the diet. Either way, you should start including nuts in your diet; they taste good and they are good for you.

Other studies of trans fats have found no evidence that trans fats can cause cancer, but they may be one of the many causes of diabetes.[48,49] Armed with this information, the Institute of Medicine has recommended that the intake of trans fats be as low as possible. The minimum amount of trans fats a person can consume and not increase risk is zero.

Where Are the Trans Fats?

If the safe recommended amount of trans fats is zero, the trans fats we currently eat should be identified and eliminated from our diets. How can you know if the food you eat has trans fats? This is where the battle for good health gets complex. Before the health risks of trans fats were known, the food industry had no reason not to use them. After decades of food development and design, many of the processed and prepackaged foods we consume are prepared with trans fats. The fast food and bakery industries depend on reliable, inexpensive frying oil to help them prepare foods. Table 7.1 shows the saturated and trans fats contents of common foods. Total fat grams is the sum of all four types of fats in a food.

Product	Common serving size	Total fat g	Sat. fat g	Trans fat g
French fries	medium	27	7	8
Butter	1 tbsp	11	7	0
Margarine, stick	1 tbsp	11	2	3
Margarine, tub	1 tbsp	7	1	0.5
Mayonnaise (soybean oil)	1 tbsp	11	1.5	0
Shortening	1 tbsp	13	3.5	4
Potato chips	small bag	11	2	3
Milk, whole	1 cup	7	4.5	0
Milk, skim	1 cup	0	0	0
Doughnut	1	18	4.5	5
Candy bar	1	10	4	3

Table 7.1 Fat content of common foods[58]

Unless the foods you eat are listed in this table, you may have no idea if they contain trans fats. Even if you look at the nutrition label, you still won't be able to determine if trans fats are included. That's because food manufacturers are currently not required to list trans fats on their food labels. As early as 1994, the FDA received formal requests that trans fats be listed, but public comment, additional research, and discussion delayed any label changes. Action on the new label requirement wasn't finalized until 2003, when the FDA gave food manufacturers until January 2006 to have their labels updated. The FDA estimates that three years after the effective date, the new labels will prevent from 600 to 1,200 heart attacks and will save 250 to 500 lives in the first year. This improvement in health will translate into a savings of $900 million to $1.8 billion per year in medical costs, lost productivity, and pain and suffering. So for now you only have two options. You can buy foods from food manufacturers that really care about your health and have already changed their labels, or you can read the ingredients and see if the food was made with trans fats. One such label looks like this:

Total Fat   6g
    Saturated Fat 0.5g
    Trans Fat   0g

As of the writing of this book, Frito-Lay has already included trans fat content on most of its brands, including Lay's, Doritos, Cheetos, Fritos, Tostitos, Ruffles, Rold Gold, and Sunchips. In fact, the fat label above is from a package of Tostitos Corn Chips. Way to go Frito-Lay! They have accepted this new requirement and have reduced or eliminated trans fats from most of their foods. This demonstrates to the public and the best nutrition experts in the world that Frito-Lay is serious about providing healthy foods.

Other food manufacturers, however, may be more concerned with profits than customer health. After all, Altria (formerly Phillip Morris) still advertises cigarettes. Like they really care about your health! Altria also owns Nabisco, which is part of Kraft Foods. Kraft Foods offers a line of food products that is full of saturated and trans fats, many of which are leaders on the saturated and trans fats list of heavy hitters.

In 2003, Kraft was threatened with a lawsuit for its aggressive promotion of Oreo cookies in the schools in California. Just a few days after the suit was announced, Kraft declared that it would reformulate the cookies and make a version without trans fats. Traditional Oreo cookies have 3.5 grams of trans fats per serving, and the new variety has no trans fats. Lawsuits can sometimes bring about needed change. Kraft has also listed trans fats on the label for its Triscuit crackers and has produced a version that is free of trans fats. Progress is being made, but a company like Kraft has a lot of work to do before its food products can really promote and not threaten health.

Much of the food industry fought against the new labels that require information about trans fats, but it appears that public health is eventually going to overcome food industry protectionism. For a rather chilling view of the aggressive tactics of the food industry, I suggest Marion Nestle's book *Food Politics.*

I predict that within the next few years, someone will sue a school district because the schools provide only unhealthy fast foods and candies in their vending machines—mostly soft drinks and foods that are high in trans fats and saturated fats. The schools maintain very lucrative contracts with the vendors, and the children at the schools are given very few healthy options from vending machines. However, because many schools are unwilling to remove the unhealthy foods for fear of losing the vending profits, they may be guilty of a failure to provide a safe school environment. Several leading pediatric medical journals have warned pediatricians about this very issue, but I'm not sure schools are able look past the money to hear the message.[59,60] I hope they start to make voluntary changes without painful and expensive litigation.

Perhaps the only group of food producers that are going to get away without a scratch are those in the fast food industry. Since the food is purchased hot, it is not required to have a nutrition label and customers will never really know about the foods' trans fats content. Think of all the fried foods in American fare: french fries, onion rings, corn dogs, popcorn, seafood, chips, and, oooh, those bakery goods. Maple bars, doughnuts, croissants, éclairs—all of them are deep fried in trans fats. The only way you would know would be if you were to see a list of the ingredients.

The food label and ingredients list included below is for an American icon—the glazed doughnut. The label shows that one doughnut has 13 grams of fat, of which 3 grams are saturated fat. So far it doesn't look really bad except that the other fat grams are not accounted for. Surely there must be some healthy fats in there, but you can't tell from the label.

The clue to this mystery is in the ingredients list. Bolded you will see "partially hydrogenated soybean and/or cottonseed oil." On another label it might say "vegetable shortening" or "partially hydrogenated vegetable oil," but this is your sign that trans fats are used to make the food. The closer it is listed to the beginning of the ingredients list, the more of it there is in the food. The ingredients for this doughnut include bleached flour, dextrose (used to get the yeast to work well), and trans fats. From Table 7.1 you can see that a simple doughnut has 5 grams of trans fats.

Take a look at the label of your favorite peanut butter. All the popular brands list trans fats in the ingredients, but the trans fat content of the peanut butter is so low that even when the new labeling requirements are

Nutrition Facts

Serving Size 1 Doughnut (52g)
Servings Per Container

Amount Per Serving

Calories 200   Calories from Fat 110

% Daily Value*

Total Fat 12g	**18%**
Saturated Fat 3g	**15%**
Cholesterol 5mg	**1%**
Sodium 95mg	**4%**
Total Carbohydrate 22g	**7%**
Dietary Fiber less than 1g	**2%**
Sugars 10g	
Protein	

Vitamin A 0%	•	Vitamin C 2%
Calcium 0%	•	Iron 4%

Ingredients: Enriched bleached wheat flour (contains bleached wheat flour, niacin, reduced iron, thiamine mononitrate, riboflavin, folic acid), dextrose, **vegetable shortening (partially hydrogenated soybean and/or cottonseed oil),** water, sugar, soy flour, egg yolks, vital wheat gluten, yeast, nonfat milk, yeast nutrients (calcium sulfate, ammonium sulfate), dough conditioners (calcium dioxide, monocalcium and dicalcium phosphate, diammonium phosphate, sodium stearoyl-2-lactylate, whey, starch, ascorbic acid, sodium bicarbonate, calcium carbonate), salt, mono- and diglycerides, ethoxylated mono-and diglycerides, lecithin, calcium propionate (to retain freshness), cellulose gum, natural and artificial flavors, fungal alpha amylase, amylase, maltogenic amylase, pentosanase, protease, sodium caseinate, corn maltodextrin, corn syrup solids and BHT (to help protect flavor).

enforced, you won't see any trans fats listed on the label.[61] The amount of trans fats in peanut butter is below the amount needed to be listed. So go ahead, smear some peanut butter on that sandwich.

McDonalds restaurants announced in 2002 that they were going to introduce a new cooking oil into all of its restaurants. The oil is supposed to have half the amount of trans fats as their previous frying oil. Two years later, the change hasn't happened. Hopefully it will.

Trading Calories

You can add more poly- and monounsaturated fats to your diet by eating more foods that contain these fats, but that would increase the number of calories you eat and possibly cause you to gain weight. Instead of adding these fats to your diet, a better way would be to substitute good fats for bad fats. The average man eats about 2,700 calories a day and the average woman eats about 1,800 calories. Most of these calories (52%) come from carbohydrates, and 14% comes from protein. The rest of the calories (34%) come from the four different fat sources. The pie chart in Figure 7.3 shows the sources of the calories we eat.

When substituting bad fats for good fats, you get a double benefit. First, trans and saturated fats would be reduced and unsaturated poly and

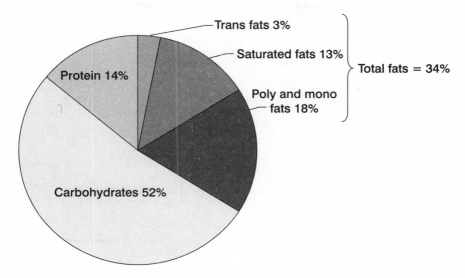

Figure 7.3 Sources of the calories we eat[12,62]

mono fats would be increased. And second, when you reduce the fats that increase your risk of chronic disease. Suppose you decided to reduce the amount of saturated fat in your diet by 5% of total calories and increase the unsaturated part by the same amount. You could do this if you avoided high-fat dairy products and fatty meats and ate more plant oils. Data from the Nurses' Health Study show that the health benefits of this substitution would reduce your chances of heart attack and death by 40%.[63] If you substituted just 2% of total calories from trans fats with the same amount of good fats, you could reduce your risk by 50%. In other words, replacing most dietary trans fats with healthy fats could potentially prevent 347,877 heart disease deaths per year.[63,64]

I do not wish to be the bearer of bad food news. On the contrary, the purpose of this book is to share with the public what researchers already know—the research that is reported in scientific journals rarely trickles down to the public unless someone puts it into understandable English and finds a way to make it applicable to real people living real lives. In that regard, I'm just a messenger.

POINTS TO REMEMBER:

- The all-fats-are-bad approach to eating may be like throwing out the baby with the bath water.

- There are both good and bad fats; the best are fats from plants and nuts and the worst are saturated and trans fats.

- Americans are eating less fat but getting more calories.

- Eliminate trans fats from your diet and try adding more healthy fats.

- Use the new food labels; they will help you avoid trans fats.

8

The Rest of the Good Nutrition Lineup

It is useless for the sheep to pass resolutions in favor of
vegetarianism while the wolf remains of a different opinion.
—William Ralph Inge (1860–1954)

SO FAR YOU HAVE LEARNED ABOUT THE BENEFITS of eating fruits, vegetables, whole grains, nuts, and healthy fats. These foods form the nutritional foundation on which you can add other healthy and delicious foods. In this chapter, we will talk about the top three layers of the healthy eating pyramid, which include meat, poultry, eggs, dairy products, refined starches, and alcohol. The best available evidence suggests foods included in these upper layers should be eaten in moderation. Unfortunately, many Americans increase their risk of chronic diseases by eating too many of these foods.

When you take a group of really smart people and pay them to come up with unique ways to identify a healthy diet, it is surprising what they can devise. Several researchers from Harvard University and from Brigham and Women's Hospital in Boston came up with a way to represent what healthy and unhealthy diets look like by identifying two distinct diet patterns. They called a healthy diet a prudent diet, and they called an unhealthy diet a Western diet. This approach to finding a healthy way to live was quite brilliant because it used data from several large cohort studies.

In identifying a healthy diet, researchers used computers and sophisticated pattern recognition techniques to identify food patterns associated
with certain diseases. For example, the researchers used diet data on 42,500
middle-aged men who had participated in the Health Professions study to
identify who might be at risk for diabetes.[1] This analysis was also conducted
in a study of women.[2] In the Harvard University and Brigham and Women's
Hospital study, the computers were programmed to consider every possible
combination of food groups, types, and categories. The result was that researchers identified two types of common food-consumption patterns. One
pattern was described as being high in red meat, processed meat, french
fries, high-fat dairy foods, refined grains, and sweets and desserts. This one
was called the "Western" pattern because it accurately described the diet
of many Americans and people who live in countries that have become
Westernized. The other common pattern included high amounts of fruits,
vegetables, whole grains, legumes, fish, poultry, and low-fat dairy products
and was called the "prudent" pattern. Which of these patterns best describes
your diet? Do you follow a prudent diet or a Western diet?

When the computer models were used to predict which individuals
might develop diabetes, these two diet patterns emerged, with women
producing the same pattern as men. Researchers determined that if you
follow a prudent diet, you have a 16% lower risk of developing diabetes, but
if you follow a Western diet, your risk increases by 59%.

Would other diseases have similar patterns or different ones? Other
researchers used the same computer technique to identify diet patterns
associated with coronary heart disease,[3-6] and the dietary patterns they
identified were almost identical to the patterns associated with diabetes. The
prudent diet was associated with a 34% reduction in risk of heart disease
and the Western diet was linked with a 64% increase in risk. These two diet
patterns were even associated with physiological changes that are believed to
cause cardiovascular disease and obesity.[7] So, now we have two very different
chronic diseases being linked with the same pattern of food intake.

You might wonder if these food patterns are also associated with other
chronic diseases like cancer or strokes. Very good! You are starting to think
like a Harvard professor. This is exactly the question Harvard researchers
asked. Teaming up with Swedish scientists, the same process was used
to identify diet patterns that might be associated with colorectal cancer.[8]
Once again, the patterns identified were almost identical to the patterns
previously connected with diabetes and heart disease. Study participants
who had prudent diets also had fewer cases of cancer. Other researchers

used these same techniques to see who might get breast cancer, but this time the patterns failed to be related to new cases of breast cancer.[9] This just shows that doing research can be very frustrating. These two diet patterns identified who might get diabetes, heart disease, and colon cancer, but failed to be associated with breast cancer. It seems to work extremely well with some chronic diseases, but not so well with breast cancer. It is surprising that even though each study used a different set of data and looked at a different disease, the overall diet patterns were strikingly similar. Each identified red meat, processed meats, and high-fat dairy foods as part of an unhealthy Western diet.

The "V" Word

INSIDE THE ALDANA HOME ►►► *I was sitting on my porch reading a book when a total stranger drove up to my house and introduced himself as someone who had read some of my research and wanted to talk to me about vegetarian diets. I would describe our conversation as a mixture of science, scripture, politics, and a well-rehearsed recounting of this man's successful cancer remission because of his newfound vegetarian lifestyle.*

After three hours the man finally left and I retired to bed. At seven o'clock the next morning he knocked on my door and presented me with an armful of books he wanted me to read. The titles included things like The Crazy Makers: How the Food Industry Is Destroying Our Brains and Harming Our Children, *and, one of my favorites,* Milk: The Deadly Poison.

That was my first experience with what I call vegetarian missionaries—a small number of individuals who have an intense desire to convert others to their vegetarian way of life. Most of these individuals have had a life-changing experience that has convinced them that their course of action changed their life, and they want others to be able to experience the same transformation.

I'm very happy when people are able to overcome serious health issues, regardless of the reason for the recovery, and I am wise enough to know that just about anything is possible. There is no way of knowing if changing to a vegetarian diet is what saved this man's life. It is possible, but studies that introduced cancer victims to healthy diets have demonstrated that diet has virtually no effect on cancer once it has spread. This man was so convinced that the new lifestyle had saved his life that he dedicated his life to spreading the life-changing effects of the vegetarian way of life. The books he left with me indicated that he was not the only one on a mission to save the world, and I can hardly blame them for being passionate. After all, the desire to help others enjoy a healthy life is the reason I wrote this book. The difference is that I have carefully reviewed every piece of scientific evidence on each aspect of nutrition and exercise and include the recommendations of the best researchers in the world—not just the ones who support my way of thinking.

Because of the experience I had with this vegetarian missionary, I became acutely aware that it is possible to scare people away from adopting healthy lifestyles. One of my fears is that the information discussed so far in this book may give you the impression that good health can be had only if you forsake all the foods you enjoy in your life. I worry that you might think you have to become a vegetarian in order to enjoy good health. I don't even like to use the "V" word because some people may have had an unpleasant experience like the one I had. Let me assure you that the information provided in this book is flexible enough to encompass a wide variety of personal food preferences, habits, and cultures, including those who wish to be vegetarians.

People choose to be vegetarians for a variety of reasons. They hope to improve their health. They may want to preserve and protect the environment. They may have compassion for animals and don't believe animals should be killed for any reason. Others are vegetarians for spiritual reasons. I like and support all of these reasons and believe there are many benefits to a vegetarian diet. However, there is ample evidence that it is not necessary to avoid all meat and dairy products in order to enjoy good health.

A healthy lifestyle can be interpreted to mean a lot of different things to different people. It is possible to have a healthy lifestyle and be a vegetarian. It is also possible to enjoy all the benefits of healthy living and not be a vegetarian. Both diets can prevent chronic diseases, and both can extend life. A discussion of the roles of meat and milk in a healthy lifestyle will help you decide which diet pattern is best for you.

Meat

The science we reviewed in our previous discussions of whole grains, fruits, vegetables, and the four different types of fats are generally in agreement on the benefits and risks associated with each of these groups as part of a healthy diet. Unfortunately, the science on the benefits of meat and milk is not quite as definitive. Extremely large databases and powerful computer modeling programs consistently identify red meat—meat from cattle, sheep, and wild game such as deer and elk—and processed meats—any meats that have been highly processed, such as hot dogs, sausage, bacon, and bologna—as being directly linked with several chronic diseases. At the same time, red meat is a good source of iron, minerals, protein, and some vitamins; it can be prepared in unlimited ways and has a taste that makes it a preferred food in the United States; and it is a traditional American food that has become part of the very fabric of American culture. It is also one of the most heavily marketed foods in America.

It's a Mixed Bag

Teasing out the effects of a single food is very difficult for researchers to do. Most often studies look at either diet patterns or specific nutrients like saturated fat or dietary cholesterol. The research on the pros and cons of meat is, therefore, difficult to conduct and different studies rarely come up with the same findings.

For example, scientists around the world have completed a total of 45 studies on meat and colorectal cancer.[10] While meat in general has not been shown to create an additional cancer risk, the studies that isolated red and processed meats indicated they may cause colorectal cancer. I use the word *may* because of the 45 published studies, 32 showed no link between meat consumption and colorectal cancer; the 13 remaining studies showed a significant link with cancer. Not a single study suggested eating meat would somehow protect against cancer.[11,12]

Studies that compared colorectal cancer rates between vegetarians and nonvegetarians detected no difference in cancer rates between the two groups.[11] If there truly were a large danger to eating meat, the results of the studies would likely be more consistent.

There are 20 studies that looked at the relationship between eating meat and breast cancer. A review of all these studies showed that they failed to link red meat, white meat, or any meat with breast cancer. These same studies also failed to show a convincing link between egg and dairy product consumption and breast cancer.[13]

Just one year after this review was published, one of the largest and best designed studies yet showed that animal fat was significantly linked with breast cancer in middle-aged women, making the evidence of a link between meat consumption and breast cancer even more difficult to understand.[14] Though these studies have failed to consistently report more risk for meat eaters, a large study of Seventh-Day Adventists, who are encouraged to be vegetarians, showed that a diet low in meat appears to increase lifespan an average of 3.6 years when compared to a diet that excluded meat.[15]

In addition to the study from the Seventh-Day Adventists, six other studies have evaluated how a low-meat diet is related to lifespan. Of these, five showed low-meat diets extended lifespan and one showed no difference.[16] (Eating meat less than weekly was the definition of low-meat intake.)

The diet-pattern studies mentioned at the beginning of this chapter all show that red meat and processed meat intake appear to be related to an increased risk of diabetes, colon cancer, and coronary heart disease. Some have suggested that this relationship is direct—the more red meat you eat, the greater your risk of these diseases.[17,18]

We can take this enormous amount of research and condense it down to the following simple statement that best describes the science today: *Red meat and processed meat probably increase the risk of cardiovascular disease and colorectal cancer; if you eat meat, you should do so sparingly.*[19] Notice on the Healthy Eating Pyramid that red meat is strategically located at the tip of the pyramid. It is there for a purpose: to show that it should be eaten sparingly. The link between meat and colorectal cancer is not well understood, but the increased risk is theorized to be due to the high saturated-fat content of red meat or to eating burned, charred meat. When meat is cooked on an open flame, excessive heat can cause proteins and sugars in the meat to form cancer-causing chemicals called heterocyclic amines. When you eat the meat, you eat the chemicals.[20,21] The chemicals then pass through your intestines and irritate your colon, which can lead to cancer.

The prudent diet pattern and the Mediterranean diet show that poultry (including eggs) and fish (when eaten in moderation) may contribute to good health. The healthy Greeks who followed a Mediterranean diet were eating zero to four eggs a week.[22] Eggs do contain cholesterol and they can cause small changes in your body's cholesterol,[23] but cohort studies of egg consumption and heart disease have failed to put eggs on the do-not-eat list.[24,25] The Healthy Eating Pyramid shows that a good diet should include zero to two servings of fish, poultry, or eggs every day.

Milk: Does a Body Good or Deadly Poison?

Few foods stir more passion, debate, anger, or emotion than milk. The role of milk in American society is defined by tradition, economics, science, and politics. You've seen the paid celebrities who have agreed to have their pictures taken with whole-fat milk coating their upper lip like a white mustache. The "Got Milk" message portrayed in these ads is that if celebrities are drinking whole milk, you and I should be drinking whole milk.

On the other end of the spectrum, certain groups have written about some of the research on milk that links milk with allergies, immune deficiencies, cancers, and a host of other chronic diseases. One author has titled his book *Milk: The Deadly Poison*. We have celebrities selling milk as the great promoter of health and, at the same time, concerned citizens labeling it a deadly poison.

In addition to these polarized opinions about milk, there are literally hundreds of studies that have looked at countless effects and benefits believed to be associated with milk consumption. Interestingly, many of these studies were funded by the dairy industry—which introduces the appearance of a conflict of interest.

Let's use the following question as an example: Does milk make strong bones? Researchers have conducted 57 different studies looking at dairy foods and bone health. Of the 57 studies, 30 showed that eating dairy foods did build strong bones, and the dairy industry was quick to tell the world that milk "does a body good." However, in another 24 of the 57 studies, eating dairy foods had no effect on bone health, and 3 of the studies found that eating dairy foods actually decreased bone health.[26] As you might expect, the anti-milk groups use these studies to support their cause.

As this example demonstrates, it doesn't really matter what opinions you may have about dairy foods; there are plenty of studies out there to support whatever health belief you may have. Therefore, the only reliable method anyone has of sorting through the fact and fiction related to milk is to rely on the overall consensus of the research because the consensus includes all completed studies—not just the ones funded by the dairy industry or other special interest groups, but every single study that has been published in a peer-reviewed journal.

Dairy products are those products that include milk as a primary ingredient. Cheese, milk, yogurt, and ice cream are the most common dairy foods we consume, all of which come in low-fat versions. Early studies of the effects of milk on health did not distinguish between high-fat and low-fat or skim milk so, unfortunately, many of the results refer to milk products in general.

The study of prudent and Western diet patterns does a nice job of highlighting the differences between high- and low-fat dairy foods and their relationships to chronic diseases. High-fat dairy foods are part of a diet that increases the risk of chronic diseases, while low-fat dairy foods seem to protect against many chronic diseases.[27] The same is true for dairy foods and cancer. Over 30 case-control and cohort studies tried to determine if dairy foods were related to colorectal cancer.[28] The cohort studies consistently showed that eating dairy foods actually decreased the risk of getting colorectal cancers, but the case-control studies found that dairy foods had no effect on these cancers. Dairy foods were also shown not to cause breast cancer.[13,29] This conclusion came from the summary of 20 different studies. About the only cancer that has any apparent association with dairy products is prostate cancer, and even this research is inconclusive; some studies show a relationship and some do not.[30-32]

Milk allergies

One common concern with drinking milk is milk allergy or allergy to dairy products. It is estimated that 2–3% of infants have an adverse reaction to cow's milk protein,[33] a reaction that can also happen with mother's milk. The most common indicator of a reaction occurs about one hour after ingesting milk, when infants have digestive distress or their skin breaks out in red splotches. Most infants who have this allergic response get it before one month of age, and although worrisome, this allergy is not life threatening, and almost all children are able to tolerate milk by the age of three. There is some evidence that children who are truly allergic to cow's milk protein or mother's milk often have other allergies.

In the late 1950s, researchers began studying the health of people in the United States, Finland, the Netherlands, Italy, the former Yugoslavia, Greece, and Japan.[34] The study was called the Seven Countries Study. Diet and cause-of-death data were tracked for 25 years and showed which countries have the highest heart disease death rates. During the time of the study, 268 out of every 1,000 people in Finland died of heart disease, but in Greece only 25 per 1,000 died of the same disease. The differences between the countries were most pronounced in the people's diets. People who ate the most butter, meat, pastries, and milk had the highest death rates—further evidence that high-fat dairy foods may be linked with chronic disease.

High-fat dairy foods contain a high percentage of saturated fat. Remember from our discussion of fats that saturated fat in high quantities increases the risk of heart disease and stroke. When high-fat dairy foods are compared to low-fat dairy foods, it looks like good health may be protected with dairy products that are low in fat; the risk of cardiovascular disease and stroke is lower for those who eat low-fat dairy products,[35,36] including skim

What is lactose intolerance?

Lactose intolerance is the inability to digest significant amounts of lactose, the predominant sugar of milk. This inability results from a shortage of the enzyme lactase, which is normally produced by the cells that line the small intestine. Lactase breaks down milk sugar into simpler forms that can then be absorbed into the bloodstream. When there is not enough lactase to digest the amount of lactose consumed, the person can experience nausea, cramps, bloating, gas, and diarrhea, which begin about 30 minutes to 2 hours after eating or drinking foods containing lactose. For most people, lactose intolerance develops naturally over time. After 2 years of age, the body begins to produce less lactase, but most people may not experience symptoms until they are much older. Between 30 and 50 million Americans are lactose intolerant. As many as 75% of all African-Americans and American Indians and 90% of Asian Americans are lactose intolerant. Those who are of a northern European descent are least likely to have the condition. There is no way to help the body produce more lactase, but by avoiding foods with lactose mainly milk, cheese, or milk products, you can avoid the symptoms. There is also a lactase pill or liquid that can be eaten with meals that contain milk products.

and 1% milk and low-fat ice cream or cheeses. A diet that includes fruits, vegetables, and low-fat dairy products can also reduce blood pressure.[37]

Figure 8.1 shows the trends in the consumption of whole milk and low-fat milk over the past 90 years. It looks like the message has been getting out: Dairy products are okay, but low-fat versions are the better choice.

Glycemic Index

In chapter 5 we talked about the antioxidants, phytochemicals, and fiber found in whole grains. There is one more reason why whole grains

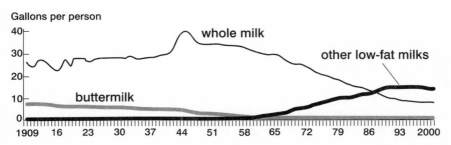

Lower fat milks include buttermilk (1.5% fat), plain and flavored reduced-fat milk (2% fat), low-fat milk (1% fat), nonfat milk, and yogurt made from these milks (except frozen yogurt).

Figure 8.1 Americans are switching to lower fat milks

may be good for you. Recall that refined white flour has had the bran and germ removed so all that is left is the starchy flour. White bread is made from bleached, refined flour. When you eat a piece of white bread, the carbohydrates in the flour are easily broken down into glucose, which is quickly absorbed through the wall of the stomach and the first part of the small intestine. As the glucose enters the bloodstream, the body senses the additional glucose and the pancreas releases insulin.

Insulin is a glucose escort. Without it, glucose cannot enter a cell because it cannot get through the cell wall. Because the digestion of white bread is so fast, there is a rapid increase in the amount of glucose that enters the bloodstream. This prompts a rapid and large release of insulin. So much insulin is released that the amount of glucose in the blood drops dramatically. The

---

The rate at which white bread is digested and absorbed into the bloodstream is called white bread's glycemic index. The value for the glycemic index of white bread is 100.

---

cells are happy because they get lots of glucose for energy, but the bloodstream is left with too little glucose, leaving you in a state of hypoglycemia, or low blood sugar. Although hypoglycemia sounds alarming, it's actually quite normal—it happens to all of us every time we feel hungry. Low blood sugar is one of the reasons we sense hunger. Different foods are absorbed at different rates; white bread is absorbed rather quickly. In fact, the rate at which the body digests white bread is the measuring stick by which the absorption rates of all other foods are determined. The rate at which white bread is digested and absorbed into the bloodstream is called white bread's glycemic index. The value for the glycemic index of white bread is 100.

Instant rice is absorbed even faster than white bread. It has a glycemic index of 124 and is considered to be a high-glycemic-index food. Table sugar has a glycemic index of 83. That's right, you read correctly; table sugar has a lower glycemic index than white bread because it takes longer to enter the bloodstream. Popcorn, fruit, vegetables, whole grains, beans, and skim milk all have indexes much lower than that of white bread.

The rate at which foods are digested is dependent on many different factors. For example, a piece of fruit has a different index depending on its ripeness—ripe fruits have a lower index. If you chew your food a lot, it will have a higher index because the smaller particles are digested more quickly. A whole apple has one index, applesauce has a different index, and apple juice has a third index. Different pastas have different values depending on the type of pasta you eat.[38] Foods that are processed or cooked more than others have a different index, so if you boil, bake, or fry something (like a potato), you will get three slightly different indices. Suppose you use white bread and make a tuna sandwich with lettuce, pickles, and mayonnaise served with fresh fruit and some chips made without trans fats. Even though the white bread has a high glycemic index, the entire meal, when eaten at one setting, actually has a low glycemic index. The way glucose is absorbed into the bloodstream is dependent on what foods are eaten at the same time.

You can see that trying to make a recommendation on which foods to eat, how to cook them, when to pick them, how to chew them, and so on and so forth, would be unrealistic. Yet that's what it would take to closely follow a low-glycemic-index diet. Until additional well-designed studies are completed, there is not enough information to make recommendations to the public. Besides, if you really think about what was presented in the last three chapters, carefully learning the glycemic index of every food you eat is rather silly. If you follow a prudent diet consisting of whole grains; fruits and vegetables; low-fat dairy products; good fats; and fish, poultry, eggs, and with red meat consumed in moderation, you are already getting a diet that has a low glycemic index.[39]

You might be wondering, why spend so much time discussing the glycemic indices of foods? Take another look at the Healthy Eating Pyramid. At the tip you will see white rice, white bread, potatoes, pasta, and sweets. These are all foods that have a high glycemic index, and they are listed at the top for that reason.

Laboratories all over the world have been carefully testing the glucose absorption properties of literally thousands of different foods. (The results of this testing can be found online at www.glycemicindex.com and in countless books that have been published on the subject.) It took a while but eventually the glycemic indices for most foods were determined. This gave scientists the ability (after surveying people about their nutrition) to calculate the glycemic index for the whole diet, an index value that represents the sum total of a person's diet. People who eat a lot of refined carbohydrates have an index higher than people who eat a more prudent diet. With index values for whole diets, researchers were finally able to determine if there was any relationship between diet, glycemic index, and many chronic diseases; it appears there is.

Weight-loss studies have shown that diets based on foods that have a low glycemic index may enhance weight control[40] because they appear to delay the onset of hunger, which in turn helps people eat less often and in smaller amounts.[41] Such diets reduce the amount of insulin that is secreted after meals, and they appear to help the body use insulin more efficiently. A few studies have shown that dieters on low-glycemic diets may even be able to lose greater amounts of weight than people who eat high-glycemic-index foods.

Remember, when a lot of glucose enters the bloodstream in a short amount of time, the pancreas has to produce large quantities of insulin. Some theorize that the insulin-producing cells get worn out. Others think that because so much insulin is produced, the body slowly stops recognizing the insulin and becomes insulin resistant. The Nurses' Health Study showed that women with a diet high in foods with a high glycemic index have a greater risk of developing diabetes, while women who consume foods with a low glycemic index have a significantly lower risk of diabetes.[42]

Foods with a high glycemic index have also been linked with cardiovascular disease.[43] The rapid influx of glucose and the subsequent rush of insulin appear to affect blood cholesterol. Low-glycemic-index foods increase good cholesterol and reduce bad cholesterol and total cholesterol. This is evidenced by the lower rates of heart disease among those who eat low-glycemic-index foods. A few case control studies have even linked high-glycemic-index foods with colon and breast cancers.[44]

When the pilgrims came to North America, they discovered Native Americans who for centuries had followed what some might consider a prudent diet. After becoming assimilated into Western culture, Native Americans abandoned their original food traditions and habits and adopted a Western diet pattern, which includes many foods with a high glycemic index. With this change in diet came a change in diseases. Native American tribes have the highest rates of diabetes in the country; the Pima Indians of Arizona have a prevalence of diabetes that is 2.6 times higher than the American population in general. Perhaps one of the best applications that will come from the glycemic index research will be to assist individuals who are diabetic.

In the past few years, inspiring authors, writers, and weight-loss entrepreneurs have taken the limited amount of science that exists on the glycemic index and attempted to revolutionize the weight-loss industry. It may well be that foods that have a low glycemic index can help with weight control, reduce the risks of diabetes and heart disease, and maybe even reduce the risk of certain cancers. It is impossible to know for sure without large, randomized clinical trials, so until then, don't worry about the whole glycemic index thing. Besides, if you are eating a prudent diet, it will never be an issue.

Can Alcohol Be Part of a Healthy Lifestyle?

Not shown in the Healthy Eating Pyramid is the current recommendation regarding the use of alcohol. When alcohol enters the bloodstream, it keeps the blood from clumping or clotting and increases the amount of good cholesterol. These two effects of alcohol keep arteries from becoming blocked, which prevents many cardiovascular diseases including heart disease and stroke, and may help prevent heart disease death.[45-47] A moderate amount of alcohol—no more than one drink per day for a woman and one to two drinks per day for a man—is enough to provide this protection. However, this is the only known health benefit of drinking.

Some may think that if a little alcohol is good, than a lot is even better, but it doesn't work that way. Figure 8.2 shows the risk of cancers and cardiovascular diseases that are associated with alcohol consumption. The numbers at the bottom of the graph are the average number of drinks per day. If you drink a small to moderate amount of alcohol (one to two drinks a day), you will actually see a slight decrease in the risk of cardiovascular disease. Abstaining from alcohol increases your risk slightly, and drinking more than a moderate amount reverses any protection you may have had and can add even more risk. The solid line in the figure shows this phenomenon, which researchers actually call a J-shaped risk curve. (I think it looks more like the swoosh found on Nike products.)

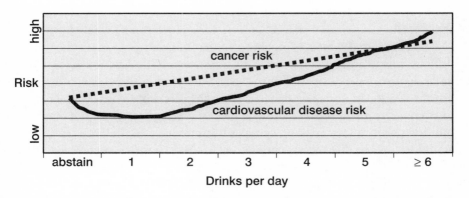

Figure 8.2 Risk of cancer and cardiovascular diseases in relation to alcohol consumption. The solid line shows the risk of cardiovascular diseases; the dotted line shows cancer risk.

Despite the documented benefit of drinking moderate amounts of alcohol, there is a whole host of reasons alcohol should be avoided or at least consumed in low amounts. The dotted line in Figure 8.2 shows how the risk of cancer increases as alcohol consumption goes up. It does not have a J shape like the line for cardiovascular disease; it is a straight, undeviating line that only goes up as the amount of alcohol consumed increases.[48]

Many very good studies have also shown that alcohol consumption is related to cancers of the throat, esophagus, rectum, liver, stomach, colon, and breast.[49,50] The more you drink, the greater your risk of developing these diseases. Low to moderate amounts of alcohol do not protect against these cancers; they actually make them slightly more likely.

Alcohol affects every organ in your body. Long-term heavy drinking can cause liver and pancreas diseases. If you are pregnant or trying to get pregnant, the safe amount of alcohol to consume is zero. Drinking alcohol while you are pregnant can cause a range of birth defects and conditions, including fetal alcohol syndrome, which includes severe physical, mental, and behavioral problems that stay with children for life.

Worse yet, alcohol is directly responsible for 30% of all highway fatalities. That means that of the 41,945 people killed driving in 2001, 12,793 are dead because someone was drinking and driving. Drinking can cause dangerous interactions with medications, social and legal problems (like family separations), and difficulty with relationships. Given the harmful side effects associated with alcohol, it is difficult to justify a recommendation that everyone should consume alcohol in moderation. A more prudent recommendation would be that if you drink, do so in moderation, and if you don't drink, don't start.

Don't Wait

Research on the health impacts of different foods is an example of how difficult it is to answer some scientific questions. Thousands of scholars and scientists have devised clever ways to study foods and chronic diseases, but the results do not always give us clear answers. Future research will add to what we've just discussed and will give us even more good information, but don't wait to start making changes until we have all the answers. If you would follow the diet recommendations in these chapters, there would be a reduction in the number of chronic diseases in the United States that would dwarf all other improvements in public health; it would literally transform the health of the nation. Add the benefits of physical activity and Americans would be the healthiest citizens in the world.

POINTS TO REMEMBER

- The best nutrition information at this time shows that red meat and processed meats appear to increase risk of cardiovascular disease and stroke and may be linked to colon cancer.

- Fish, poultry, and eggs can be part of a healthy lifestyle.

- Don't roll your eyes at vegetarians; they're also getting great health benefits.

- Dairy products that are low in fat should be favored over those that are high in fat.

- Forget about the glycemic index if you are planning on eating a prudent diet.

- If you drink any alcohol, do so in moderation.

CARDIORESPIRATORY FITNESS ▸

MUSCLE STRENGTH ▸

ENDURANCE ▸

FLEXIBILITY ▸

BODY COMPOSITION ▸

ENERGY ▸

SLEEP ▸

MOOD IMPROVEMENT ▸

SELF-ESTEEM ▸

SELF-CONFIDENCE ▸

SELF-CONCEPT ▸

9

What Exercise Will Do for You

A bear, however hard he tries,
grows tubby without exercise.
—*Pooh's Little Instruction Book*

I F YOU LIVED IN THE 1800S, your day probably began when you prepared your morning meal. To prepare your food, you had to first gather
a fuel, such as wood or coal, and then get the fire started. Heavy containers of water were carried from rivers, cisterns, or a nearby well if you
were lucky. Once finished with breakfast, your work day likely included a
lot of physical activity because most jobs of that time were connected with
agriculture and involved long days of hard physical labor. Even at the end of
the day, there were more chores to do and meals to prepare. Time for leisure
or relaxation was available only after all other work was completed.

If it were possible to somehow pluck some people out of the 1800s and
transport them forward to our day, they would likely be shocked at the sights
and sounds around them. They would see automobiles drive by, planes
soaring overhead—they would see strange sights in every direction.

What would they think of a fitness center? Peering through the window,
they would see people walking or jogging on moving platforms that go
nowhere. They would see rowing machines and bicycles that are fantastic
but do not move. Strangest of all might be the way people are repeatedly

lifting very heavy plates of steel, as if they were being punished or were slaves. Clearly, our world has changed.

Today we have incredible laborsaving devices. We no longer need to gather wood or start a fire to prepare our food; we simply place it in the microwave and push the button. We wash and dry our clothes with ease. There is no need for a barn for the horses; we have garages for the cars we drive and a nifty remote-control device that automatically opens and closes the door to the garage so we don't have to get out of our cars.

We go to great lengths to avoid exercise. (How many times have you gone to a store and driven around the parking lot several times in order to find the parking stall closest to the door you wish to enter?) In some ways, we have come full circle in our culture. We have done such a good job of avoiding physical labor that we now must make a special effort to get enough activity just to avoid debilitating diseases.

A lifestyle of regular physical activity can provide a wide variety of physical, mental, and social benefits. Of all the health behaviors we engage in, getting regular exercise is perhaps the hardest to commit to and maintain, yet it has tremendous benefits. Before we begin talking about starting or maintaining your own schedule of daily physical activity, you should know what's in it for you. If you already participate in regular activity, you already get the benefits; if you don't but are planning to start, you'll find out how your life can be different and what benefits you can expect.

Who Exercises?

In recent years, participation in regular physical activity has become a notable part of our society. Every day, we see people walking, jogging, bicycling, and playing organized sports. It would appear that there are more people exercising today than ever before. Unfortunately, this impression is not quite correct. As of 2000, almost 80% of all Americans are at risk for health problems because they do not get enough physical activity.[1]

If people aren't physically active in their leisure time, it is unlikely they will be physically active at other times of the day. National surveys[2] of physical activity have shown that the percentage of Americans who engage in leisure-time physical activity has remained fairly constant over the past 12 years despite government efforts to encourage physical activity (Figure 9.1), although a slight improvement was detected in the last two years of data collection. Even though the data shows that most of us are getting some leisure activity, only 20% get enough to get health benefits.

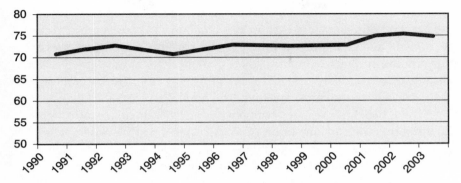

Figure 9.1 Percentage of Americans who participate in leisure-time physical activity

Children and college-age adults are more active than older adults. They tend to walk to classes, play sports and games, and participate in active recreational activities. As age increases, there is a dramatic, long-term decrease in regular physical activity. This decrease starts when most young adults begin full-time work, get married, and start families, and it continues into old age—but it doesn't have to happen. The amount of physical activity required to receive health benefits may not be as great as previously thought. For those who struggle to make exercise part of their daily lives, there are ways to make exercise more appealing and enjoyable.

A Few Terms

Physical fitness refers to how hard and how long our bodies can perform physical work and play. The health-related components of fitness include cardiorespiratory fitness, body composition, flexibility, and muscle strength and endurance. Each fitness component has a distinct effect on physical health and well-being. Some of these effects include increased endurance, decreased fatigue, decreased risk of certain cancers and cardiovascular diseases, decreased risk of obesity and subsequent diabetes, decreased chance of osteoporosis, improved sleep, and a host of other physical and emotional benefits. Physical fitness also includes characteristics such as power, agility, balance, coordination, reaction time, and speed, all of which are important for skill acquisition and sport performance but do not influence health.

Many people get adequate exercise by playing competitive sports. They like to compete and enjoy the activity and may pay little attention to the health benefits they receive. Unfortunately, some people have shied away from exercise because they think they need to be great athletes to get any benefits—that notion is not true. Not all highly trained competitors are physically fit. Some excellent golfers and baseball players are actually overweight and lack good cardiorespiratory endurance. Some athletes are outstanding performers but have diets that put them at substantial risk for chronic diseases. Other athletes focus so much of their lives on training that they may neglect the social, spiritual, and mental aspects of their lives.

Health benefits associated with physical activity do not require high-intensity training and long hours of practice. Lifetime fitness is built on physical activities that are enjoyable, easy to do, and of moderate intensity—any activity that requires you to move your body around by contracting and relaxing your muscles. However, you need to remember that it is also possible to be physically active and still not have good fitness. For example, if you walk around an office all day, you are getting physical activity and you are burning calories, but the intensity of the activity is not high enough to give you good cardiorespiratory fitness; you would still become breathless after carrying large objects or walking up a flight of stairs.

To obtain cardiorespiratory fitness, a person needs to participate in activities intense enough to cause the body to adapt to the increased physical demands and become more efficient. Fitness is determined by the intensity of the activity. The higher the intensity, the more fit you will become. All physical activity provides some health benefits, but with increased intensity, benefits also increase.

In this chapter we will focus only on the health-related components of fitness. If you are interested in improving your sport performance, seek out the advice and training of a qualified instructor or coach. Sports participation may not be for everyone, but for many, playing sports is a great way to receive good health benefits while having fun in active competition.

Cardiorespiratory Endurance

Of the four health components of physical fitness, cardiorespiratory endurance is the most important; it has the greatest impact on health. The term *cardiorespiratory endurance* refers to two important aspects of fitness: functioning of the heart (*cardio-*) and functioning of the respiratory system (*-respiratory*)—including the lungs and the veins and arteries of the body. *Cardiorespiratory endurance* and *fitness* can mean the same thing. They both refer to the ability of the heart, lungs, and vessels to provide fuel and oxygen to the body in an efficient manner.

The heart is the pump that drives the blood through the veins, arteries, and respiratory system. The volume and speed at which oxygen is delivered to the working muscles is determined by the size of the heart and the rate at which it contracts. Breathing draws oxygen into the lungs and down the bronchial tubes. These tubes lead to small ducts surrounded by capillaries. From the capillaries, oxygen from the air we breathe is transferred into the blood and carbon dioxide is released in the air we breathe out. Blood that passes through the lungs becomes rich with oxygen and is transported to all cells of the body. Once inside the cell, oxygen is used to convert the food we eat into energy (glucose) that the cells can use. Your muscles need both glucose and oxygen to do work.

Physical activity is any activity that requires you to move your body around by contracting and relaxing your muscles. Fitness is determined by the intensity of the activity. The higher the intensity, the more fit you will become.

At rest and during low-intensity physical activity, the oxygen demands of the muscles are easily met; normal breathing and a resting heart rate are enough to supply all the oxygen your body needs. If you have ever been hiking, running, or walking up a long flight of stairs, you have felt your heart and lungs working hard. You can feel your heart beating in your chest and feel the pulse in your arms and head. You notice that your breathing increases and becomes deeper. Both the amount of blood the heart pumps per beat and the rate at which the heart beats increase in proportion to the amount of work being performed. As soon as the activity stops, the muscles' demand for oxygen decreases, and the heart rate quickly returns to normal.

When each part of the cardiovascular system functions efficiently, muscle cells get enough oxygen to continue doing high amounts of work for long periods of time. In daily life, a high level of cardiorespiratory fitness gives you the ability to work and play hard without becoming fatigued or short of breath. Those who have good cardiorespiratory endurance receive many other less-obvious health benefits you are about to discover.

Body Composition

The composition of your body can be classified into two parts: lean body mass and fat. Lean body mass includes bones, muscles, organs, and connective tissue. Fat includes all the fat in your body. Some of this fat is found in and around the various organs of your body, between your skin and muscles, and inside your muscles. The amount of fat you have can be measured several ways, including the skinfold technique and underwater weighing. In chapter 4 you assessed your body weight by calculating your Body Mass Index. Body Mass Index is not a direct measure of body fat, but rather an estimation. As you already know, a certain amount of fat is essential for good health, but too much fat is unhealthy. You can improve the composition of your body by decreasing the amount of fat, increasing the amount of lean body mass, or both. Balanced nutrition keeps off excess fat, and exercise helps burn off fat and put on muscle. Increased muscle mass has the added benefit of increasing your resting metabolic rate, which means your body burns more calories even while you are at rest. This, too, helps you control and maintain a healthy weight.

Flexibility

Flexibility is the ability to move a joint through its full range of motion. When muscles and connective tissues tighten and shorten from inactivity or disuse, the range of motion in the joints is restricted. This makes it difficult to do such simple tasks as turning around in a car seat to check traffic or picking something up off the floor. On the other hand, joints that are too loose can cause you to slip or fall, to become injured, or possibly to dislocate a joint. Strengthening muscles around a loose joint helps stabilize it. Individuals who enjoy good flexibility enjoy freedom of movement, less risk of muscle or joint injury, and decreased risk of lower back pain.

Muscular Strength and Endurance

Muscular strength and endurance describes the different ways muscles are used. If you have good muscular endurance, your muscles can hold a moderately heavy weight for a long time or lift the weight repeatedly without tiring. Carrying an infant or carrying a suitcase for an extended period of time are examples of muscular endurance.

Muscular strength refers to the muscle's ability to exert maximal force. If you have ever lifted something very heavy, you have used muscular strength. The maximum amount of weight you can lift one time is a measure of muscular strength. Depending on the amount of weight you lift and the number of times you lift it, weight training exercises can develop both muscular strength and endurance. Even if you never step foot in a weight room, you can still develop some muscular strength and endurance.

Push-ups, sit-ups, and pull-ups are great activities for developing and maintaining good muscle strength and endurance.

Most individuals lift weights for two main reasons: to change the way their bodies look and to gain or maintain muscle strength. Other benefits have an even greater influence on your health and include less fatigue during regular activity, an increased ability to do work, a reduced risk of injury, and a reduced risk of back injury and pain.

What's in It for You?

The benefits of being physically active are available to those who accumulate 30 minutes of moderate-intensity physical activity most days of the week. What do you get for your 30-minute investment? Perhaps the greatest and most important benefit is a dramatically reduced risk of cardiovascular diseases. It is estimated that most deaths from cardiovascular diseases could be prevented if Americans would participate in physical activities on a regular basis. Exercise can also prevent diabetes, weight gain, certain cancers, and osteoporosis and can provide numerous other benefits. The disease-preventing benefits of physical activity are only part of the benefits package exercisers enjoy.

Prevent Cardiovascular Disease

If you aren't physically active, you are considered sedentary, and you will most likely have a low fitness level. If you exercise every day and participate in moderate physical activity, you will have a good fitness level. If you compare the long-term health of people who have low fitness with those who have high fitness, an amazingly consistent finding appears. The risk of heart disease, heart disease death, and stroke drops dramatically with increased physical activity and increased fitness.[3,4]

A summary of 67 research articles shows that people who have low fitness are two to eight times more likely to have a heart attack and are almost 30% more likely to have a stroke.[5,6] Even small increases in physical activity or fitness translate into large decreases in risk. If you are sedentary and become active and maintain that activity, you could experience a very large reduction in your risk of cardiovascular disease. This is great news for all the couch potatoes in America. If you can get moving, you can make a huge long-term improvement in your health.

This research also suggests that it is not possible to determine if this health protection is due to the physical activity or to the improvement in fitness that results from physical activity. Is it due to just moving around and burning up calories? Or is it due to the physiological changes that occur in the body as fitness increases?

It is not just cardiovascular disease that is prevented with exercise. One large study looked at fitness and people who died from different causes such as cardiovascular disease and cancer,[7] and showed that low levels of fitness are associated with increased risk of death. Sedentary individuals are eight times more likely to die from cardiovascular disease and five times more likely to die from cancer than people who have high levels of fitness. This is true for both men and women (see Figure 9.2). As your fitness level increases, the risk of death decreases rapidly at first and continues gradually decreasing until you reach a high level of fitness. Other researchers have reported similar findings.[8]

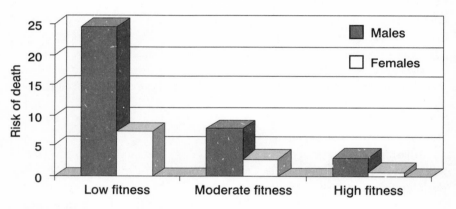

Figure 9.2 Fitness levels and risk of death from all causes

Researchers at Stanford measured the cardiorespiratory endurance of 6,000 men who had cardiovascular disease.[9] After six years, 1,256 of the men had died. When the researchers looked at high blood pressure, high blood cholesterol, body fat, fitness level, and other cardiovascular risk factors, they found a surprising result: the best predictor of death is lack of fitness.

The health-promoting effects of physical activity are not confined to those individuals who have high levels of fitness. In fact, the greatest benefit is attained when people with low fitness levels become active and improve their fitness. For example, if you were a couch potato and decided to go for a one- to two-mile walk every day, your fitness level would increase from low to moderate. If you decided to walk a little faster and go a little further, say three miles a day, you eventually would have a high level of fitness and experience an even larger drop in the risk of cardiovascular disease and certain cancers. You can achieve a high level of fitness with 30 minutes of moderate-intensity activity every day. When high levels of fitness are accompanied by reductions in cholesterol, blood pressure, smoking, and body fat, even greater decreases in death rates occur.

When you exercise, your vessels get fit. This, along with a rejuvenated heart, results in reduced blood pressure.

The reduced risk of cardiovascular disease is caused by several physiological changes that occur when the body becomes accustomed to regular physical activity. Like skeletal muscle, the heart becomes stronger with exercise. The wall of the heart thickens, and the volume of blood pumped with each contraction increases. The increased volume means the heart pumps more blood with each beat or the same amount of blood with fewer beats. This improved pumping efficiency eases the workload of the heart, and the heart beats more slowly.

The average healthy heart has a resting heart rate of 70 to 80 beats per minute (bpm). Participation in regular exercise drops the resting heart rate by 10 to 20 bpm or more. Resting heart rate is influenced not only by the strength of the heart muscle, but also by the efficiency of other parts of the circulatory system. When the entire system is functioning properly, resting heart rates can be as low as 50 to 60 beats per minute. Really fit individuals can have resting heart rates in the low 40s.

Exercise also increases the number of capillaries in the body. More capillaries mean better oxygen and carbon dioxide exchange between the blood and cells. It also means that blood flow blocked by a damaged or diseased artery can be more easily rerouted to nearby capillaries, thus avoiding serious tissue damage. Therefore, if a fit individual experiences a heart attack, it is typically less severe and recovery is faster because the blood that feeds the heart has more paths it can follow. And in the brain, a greater network of arterial capillaries helps prevent stroke, and if a stroke does occur, it is much less severe.[10] Development of this backup system of capillaries occurs in all the arteries of the body, not just the heart and brain.

Another change that occurs with physical activity affects the flow of blood. When you exercise, your blood pressure rises because your heart contracts more often and pushes an increased flow of blood through your arteries. Healthy arteries stretch and can handle the extra blood flow without any problem, so blood pressures stay in a healthy range even with the increased volume of blood. The arteries of sedentary individuals tend to become more rigid and less flexible; as a result, additional blood flow causes blood pressures to increase. Regular exercise helps keep the arteries pliable and blood pressures lower.[11]

Exercise also strengthens the muscles that help you breathe and increases the amount of air you can breathe into and out of your lungs. This means your body can remove more oxygen from the air and make it more readily available to muscles so they can do more activity. When you get fit, your heart, vessels, and respiratory system get stronger, are able to work harder, and just seem to work better.

A prime risk factor for cardiovascular disease is high blood cholesterol. Cholesterol is composed of three main parts—good cholesterol (HDL), bad cholesterol (LDL), and triglycerides. HDL helps carry fat out of the bloodstream, preventing it from forming plaque along the arterial walls, while LDL is partially responsible for the formation of fat deposits in the arteries. Regular exercise can change the proportion of these components by causing the amount of good cholesterol to increase and the amount of triglycerides to decrease. One goes up, the other goes down—but total cholesterol doesn't change, even though you have more good cholesterol.[12,13]

High blood pressure is another cardiovascular disease predictor. It doesn't matter if you begin with high blood pressure or not; when you exercise, your vessels get fit, and this, along with a rejuvenated heart, results in reduced blood pressure. The first line of treatment for high or even slightly high blood pressure is lifestyle change.[14] Fifty-five randomized clinical trials show that exercise causes a reduction in both systolic and diastolic blood pressure.[15] The higher your blood pressure when you start making lifestyle changes, the further your blood pressure will fall.[16] If your blood pressure is still high after adopting a healthy lifestyle, you should see your doctor about blood pressure medication.

There is also a close relationship between cardiovascular disease and diabetes; most diabetics die of heart disease. The first line of defense against developing diabetes is regular exercise and weight control.[17] If you are close to becoming diabetic, exercise can keep you from developing it. If you are already diabetic, exercise can improve your body's ability to recognize insulin and help your body be more sensitive to insulin when it is released into the bloodstream.[18]

SCIENCE MADE SIMPLE ▸▸▸ *When I ask people what benefits they think they get from regular physical activity, the most common response I hear is, "I feel like I have more energy." This is an interesting statement. When you exercise, you expend energy in the form of calories, you make your muscles work, and you apply stress to your bones and joints. You might expect to feel tired. However, when it comes to physical activity, it's like filling your car with gas, driving around town all day, and, at the end of the day, checking your gas gauge and finding you actually have more gas in your tank than when you started. People expend energy doing physical activity and feel like they have more energy? Strange, yes, but luckily there is an explanation for this.*

Every cell in the body has a bean-shaped organelle called a mitochondrion—the cell's power plant. It takes glucose and oxygen from the blood and converts them into a form of energy called adenosine triphosphate (ATP), the basic energy used in the body. When you exercise, your cells need more ATP to keep up with the demand for muscle movement. Since the demand for ATP is greater than the supply, shortages appear. Inside your cells, all the different parts of the cell complain and communicate about the lack of energy they are experiencing. It is like an inconvenient "power outage." The cell quickly initiates a predetermined plan and creates additional power plants to keep up with the increased demand.[19]

Power plants aren't the only part of the cell's energy utility that expands. Suppliers of energy are also affected: the number of enzymes available for transporting fat increases, and fat is more easily removed from storage and converted into energy. This is important for individuals who want to reduce body fat. If you look at muscle cells under a microscope, cells from people who are fit are dotted with more mitochondria than are cells from individuals who are sedentary. Once the cellular utility grid expands, ATP is produced at a higher rate. It is available faster and in larger amounts,[20] and everyone is happy because the energy supply has been increased.

A sedentary person who begins an exercise program can experience changes in as little as six weeks. The changes that occur in the cells go undetected. The only way you even know anything has changed is when you begin to feel like you have more energy. It's as if your gas tank got bigger and the gas works better.

Exercise Is Critical to Maintaining Healthy Body Weight

One of the most important and popular benefits of exercise is weight control and maintenance. The Healthy Eating Pyramid is constructed on a foundation of regular exercise and weight control. Weight control without regular exercise is not only nearly impossible to achieve, but it is also not advised. Chapter 12 is devoted to weight control and maintenance. Much of that chapter is devoted to the role exercise plays in both weight loss and maintenance.

Prevent Certain Cancers

Men and women who exercise regularly have a 30–40% reduction in the risk of colon cancer.[21] It seems odd that the best prevention of colon cancer that we know of comes from regular physical activity, not diet. How exercise protects against colon cancer is still unknown, but there are a few tantalizing theories.[22] Research shows that the more time food spends in the colon, the higher the risk of colon cancer. Digested food passing through the colon has constant contact with the intestinal wall, which can irritate the intestinal wall and cause lesions associated with the initial stages of cancer. Physically active individuals have a shorter transit time (food passes through the colon faster), and there is less contact with the intestinal wall. Exercisers have to go to the restroom sooner after a meal than non-exercisers. This is one explanation for physical activity protecting against colon cancer. Other researchers think that colon cancer risk is reduced because exercise improves the body's immune system and insulin sensitivity and may affect many of the hormones produced by the body. Most likely the reason for the protection is a combination of the ideas suggested in several theories.[23]

Figure 2.1 in chapter 2 shows all the studies that have looked at the relationship between breast cancer and physical activity. Not all the studies showed a protective effect from exercise, but out of 34 studies, 2 found no relationship, and 6 showed that exercise may cause breast cancer, while 26 showed that regular exercisers had 30–40% lower risk of getting breast cancer.[24] Like colon cancer, we don't have a clue why exercise is able to reduce the risk of breast cancer. A similar number of studies have been completed on other types of cancers. These reveal that physical activity doesn't cause cancer, nor does it provide any protection against cancer, except for colon and breast cancers.[21]

Many people have speculated that since physical activity can protect against certain cancers, maybe it could help cure cancer. No studies have attempted to answer this question, so the long-term benefits and risks of physical activity in cancer patients and survivors remain unknown.[25]

Build Strong Bones

SCIENCE MADE SIMPLE ▶▶▶ *Earlier we discussed the dangers associated with obesity. However, there is at least one morsel of good news floating in the sea of health risks caused by obesity. If you are obese or even overweight, you most likely have strong bones, which will protect you against osteoporosis. Your bones actually get stronger when you carry around extra weight because the weight stresses your bones and causes your body to deposit more bone mass.*

Bone is like a bank that stores bone mass. When we are young, regular exercise and adequate calcium intake make deposits in the bone bank; with every deposit, the bones get stronger. At about age 35, the withdrawals start to equal the deposits. Around age 40, your body starts to make more regular withdrawals from the bank. After menopause, withdrawals get larger every year and women can lose as much as 1–3% of their bone mass. Too many withdrawals can eventually weaken a bone enough to make it crack or collapse.

Elderly women are especially at risk for broken hips and wrists. Many women who have experienced a broken hip say that they fell and broke their hip. In reality, decades of bone withdrawals weakened the bone so much that when they were stepping up a stair or carrying a heavy object, the hip broke under the strain and they fell to the floor. In many cases, the fall does not cause the break—the bone breaks and then they fall.

If carrying extra weight increases bone mass, making your bones "think" they are carrying extra weight will have the same effect. Regular physical activity that involves weight bearing helps your body make more deposits in the bone bank and reduces the number of withdrawals.[26] This keeps the bone bank strong and almost eliminates the risk of osteoporosis. Every time you go for a walk, jog, or lift weights, your bones feel the effects of your body weight and the force of gravity. (Swimming is one of the few activities where you don't carry your body weight.)

In addition to treating osteoporosis, exercise impacts bone mass throughout life. It maximizes the amount of bone in the bone bank during youth. It maintains bone mass and slows bone loss in midlife. It preserves muscle mass and posture to reduce the risk of falls and fractures in later life.[27] If you have osteoporosis, you should engage in regular physical activity, avoid using tobacco, consume adequate dietary calcium and vitamin D, and work with your physician to determine if medication is needed. There are several safe and effective medications currently available to help combat loss of bone mass.[28]

Other Benefits

The benefits we've discussed so far are all related to common physical diseases. Regular physical activity can also impact the mental and emotional aspects of your life and improve your quality of life. It can relieve symptoms of depression and anxiety, improve mood, and may even reduce the risk of developing depression.[30] Regular physical activity is a common treatment

---

Weightlessness is bones' worst enemy

An extreme example of the opposite of weight-bearing activities is what occurs in astronauts who work for extended periods in a weightless environment. While in space, the bones of astronauts are under very little weight stress, and they lose bone mass at an alarming rate. We may have space craft that can get to Mars, but unless we figure out how to keep astronauts from losing too much bone mass, their bones would not support their weight once they reach a planet with gravity.[29]

---

for many forms of depression and may play an important role in the management of mental health diseases. Exercisers are significantly less likely to suffer from depression and other psychological disorders, including social phobias and panic or anxiety attacks.[31]

Lifting weights can reduce the symptoms of depression, put you in a better mood, and improve your self-esteem and self-confidence.[32,33] Active individuals tend to feel better about themselves and tend to have a better appearance and self-concept. Exercise can change the way you look, and if you like the way you look, you are more likely to like yourself.

Regular physical activity can impact the mental and emotional aspects of life and improve your quality of life. Exercise is like a combination of psychotherapy, physical therapy, and stress management—all concentrated in one 30-minute session.

Exercise can reduce the symptoms of stress as well as the perception of stress. Physically active people also cope with chronic and short-term stress better than those who are sedentary. A review of 34 studies showed that sedentary individuals who started engaging in physical activity had a more subdued response to stressful situations; stressful events didn't upset them as much.[34]

A commonly held belief is that regular exercise improves the quality of sleep. If you ask people who are fit if exercise helps them sleep better, most will probably say yes. To document this effect, precise measures of both exercise and sleep quality have to be used in a controlled research environment. This has been a difficult task for researchers. The best study to date showed that exercise was beneficial for individuals with sleep disorders.[35] However, a review of all existing exercise and sleep research failed to show that exercise improves sleep.[36]

 INSIDE THE ALDANA HOME ▶▶▶ *This book emphasizes the ability of science to answer important questions and guide our understanding of the requirements for healthy living. I believe in the merits of science, but I also believe there is a limit to what science can do. For example, I like to jog every morning. When I am exercising alone, I often get ideas and discover solutions to problems I've been thinking about. My run helps me clear my mind; it helps me view things from a different perspective. Many times when I arrive home, I have to quickly write down my new ideas or insights. I get mental benefits from exercise, but there is no research to document what I experience. I enjoy all the health benefits that come with exercise, but I really like the intangible ones, the ones that can't be measured.*

Exercise gives me a chance to be outside, breathe fresh air, see a little nature, and reduce my stress. Exercise is like a combination of psychotherapy, physical therapy, and stress management—all concentrated in one 30-minute session. On the days I exercise, I feel better at work, and my body doesn't feel sluggish or tired. Like many others, I feel like I have more energy. All of this adds to the total quality of my life.

I also frequently go for a walk or bike ride with my wife or children. These are great times to socialize and discuss ideas and family concerns. (Later in the book we will talk about finding time to be active.) I enjoy being with my children as we do yard work, garden, clean the garage, or even do housework; I get to spend time with my children, and we get a little exercise too.

All the health benefits discussed so far are not available solely to humans. Your pets need exercise too. Walking your dog gives both of you better health, quality time together, and a chance to be outside.

Lastly, one of the best reasons to participate in physical activity is that it is fun. Riding a bike, whacking a golf ball 250 yards down the fairway, digging in the garden, playing with children, playing sports, or just walking around can all be enjoyable. If you participate in activities that you like to do, you can have fun and improve your health at the same time.

Are You Getting the Benefits?

How can you tell if your current level of physical activity allows you to experience all the benefits we've discussed? There are two ways to do this. One way is to assess how much physical activity you get, and the other way, which is more precise, is to estimate your current fitness level. To find out if you get enough physical activity, answer yes or no to the following question: *Do you accumulate at least 30 minutes of moderate-intensity physical activity on most, preferably all, days of the week?* If you answered yes, you most likely get most of the benefits of physical activity. If you answered no, well, you and 80% of Americans should carefully study the next two chapters: "Physical Activity Nuts and Bolts" and "Being Physically Active for Life." They are written to help you become physically active and stay active for the rest of your life. The other way to determine if you are getting the benefits requires a little more work. It estimates your fitness level by how long it takes you to walk or jog 1.5 miles.

1.5-Mile Fitness Test

Figure 9.2 shows the relationship between risk of death and fitness level. To get a precise measure of fitness, you would have to take a maximal treadmill test, which accurately determines your fitness by measuring the maximum amount of oxygen you can use. During this kind of test, an exercise physiologist or cardiologist captures all the air you breathe while you walk or jog on a treadmill. The treadmill starts off slowly and gradually goes faster and faster until you can no longer keep up. Just before you have to stop, the amount of oxygen you use is measured. This method of measuring fitness is extremely accurate, but it is also very difficult for many people to do. Walking or running until you can no longer keep up can be strenuous and even dangerous for individuals who have spent a lifetime being sedentary.

The 1.5-mile fitness test does not require maximal effort, but it can still determine if you are in the low, moderate, or high fitness level.[37] To see if your fitness level is high enough to get health benefits, take the test below. It takes about 20 minutes, and it's not very hard.

Under certain circumstances, there is some risk associated with exercise. People with chronic health problems, such as heart disease, diabetes, or obesity, or who are at high risk for these problems should first obtain medical clearance from a physician before beginning a new program of physical activity. For most individuals, however, clearance to participate in low- to moderate-intensity activity can be attained by answering a few medical clearance questions. Ask yourself the following:

Has your physician ever said you have heart trouble?

Do you frequently have pains in your heart or chest?

Do you often feel faint or have spells of severe dizziness?

Do you have high blood pressure?

Has your physician ever told you that you have a bone or joint problem that is aggravated or made worse by exercise?

Is there a good medical reason why you should not engage in physical activity?

If you answered yes to any of these six questions, you should check with your doctor before proceeding. If you answered no to all six questions or you have attained medical clearance from your physician, you can take the fitness test and start moderate-intensity physical activity.

Couch potato medical clearance

Medical clearance is important if you want to prevent serious health problems. I've been asking these medical clearance questions for years, and I've never had a single person experience serious health problems because they were participating in moderate-intensity physical activity. In fact, I believe the medical clearance questions to participate in exercise are actually the wrong questions to ask. To prevent serious health problems, you should ask yourself the following questions instead:

Do you hate to exercise and avoid all physical activity or physical labor?

Do you intend to be sedentary for the rest of your life?

Are you content to be overweight and obese?

Do you currently suffer from "I-don't-care-itis"? (See chapter 3.)

If you answered yes to any of these questions, you should schedule an appointment with your physician and obtain his or her medical permission to remain sedentary. After all, if medical clearance is important to avoid putting your health at risk, anyone who answers these questions with a yes is putting their health at risk and should let their physician know.

Fitness Assessment

This test helps you determine if your fitness is sufficient to provide you with health benefits.

STEP 1: Based on your own perceived ability to cover the 1.5-mile distance, decide if you would like to walk, jog, or run the 1.5-mile distance. This is not a race; sprinting at the finish will actually give you a less accurate score. Try to maintain a constant pace. Follow the corresponding instructions below.

> *Walking instructions:* Walk at a brisk, steady pace. Slow down if you become winded.

> *Jogging instructions:* Jog at a steady, comfortable pace. Slow down or begin to walk if you become winded. Do not sprint at the end of the test—maintain a constant jogging pace the entire time.

> *Running instructions:* Run at a steady, fast pace. Slow down or begin to jog if you become winded.

STEP 2: Go to a standard track. Standard tracks are one-fourth of a mile long. You will need to complete six laps for 1.5 miles.

STEP 3: Warm up for 5 to 10 minutes. Begin when you are ready. Use a stopwatch or wristwatch to time how long it takes you to cover the distance. Don't worry if you begin jogging but find that you can't continue your pace the entire time and need to walk.

STEP 4: Record your time and consult the fitness rating table below.

Total Time (min:sec): _____

Total time (min:sec)	Fitness level	Recommendation
>19 minutes	low	Improvement recommended
12–19 minutes	moderate	You get some of the benefits
<12 minutes	high	You get most of the benefits

These fitness levels are the same ones shown in Figure 9.2. See where your fitness level is on the graph. It shows what your risk is.

POINTS TO REMEMBER

- Get more physical activity; your endurance will increase and your body will change.

- With physical activity comes protection against heart disease, stroke, diabetes, and certain cancers.

- By getting regular, moderate-intensity physical activity you can reduce your risk of premature death and chronic disease.

- Any increases in physical activity provide benefits, especially for those who are sedentary.

- Get physically active and you will help keep your bones strong, help prevent depression, and experience an improved quality of life.

- Accumulate 30 minutes or more of moderate-intensity physical activity on most, preferably all, days of the week.

FREQUENCY ▶

INTENSITY ▶

TIME ▶

MAXIMUM HEART RATE (MAX HR) ▶

TALK TEST ▶

MEDICAL CLEARANCE ▶

WARM-UP ▶

COOL DOWN ▶

CLOTHES ▶

SHOES ▶

CHAPTER 10

Physical Activity Nuts and Bolts

I believe every human has a finite number of heartbeats.
I don't intend to waste any of mine running around doing exercises.
—Neil Armstrong

"**H**OW LONG DO I HAVE TO DO THIS?**"** is one of the most common questions I am asked when I teach people about becoming physically active. I get the impression that many people feel that participating in physical activity is like taking medication: you have a health condition that needs treatment, a doctor prescribes medication, and you take the medication for a period of time until the condition goes away. For individuals who already have cardiovascular disease, exercise is a lot like a medication. It is prescribed as rehabilitation to help the heart heal and improve. Unfortunately, only 15–20% of individuals who survive a heart attack actually participate in exercise as part of their rehabilitation.[1] Most have a heart procedure and go home to live their lives just as they did before their heart attack.

Exercise is not like eating. If you don't eat, you will die within a few weeks. If you don't drink water, you will die even sooner. If you don't exercise, though, you are not necessarily going to die anytime in the near future. However, as your body adjusts to your sedentary lifestyle and metabolism, it changes in ways that foster the development of chronic diseases. In other words, a sedentary lifestyle promotes disease processes that eventually lead to premature death.

The best answer to "how long" is to ask another question: "Do you want to live a long, high-quality life or are you content to have a premature death?" To enjoy all the benefits of physical activity, you need to adopt and maintain a lifestyle of regular physical activity *for the rest of your life*. That sounds like a pretty tall order, but everyone, regardless of age, gender, race, or place of residence, can integrate physical activity into everyday living. If extending your life isn't enough to motivate you, remember that physical activity is also one half of the recipe you need to control your weight.

How Much Exercise Is Enough?

If you participate in physical activity that is planned, structured, and occurs on a repetitive basis, you are getting what is defined as exercise. Exercise is a form of structured physical activity. For many people, an exercise program helps them keep their time and life structured. Regular exercise is a great way for them to receive health benefits by participating in physical activity at a specific time and place.

When some people hear the term *exercise*, they are automatically disinterested. It's true that exercise and fitness, as described in chapter 9, are related to physical activity, but they are not necessarily the only way to obtain good health. Regardless of what you call it, the idea is to use the muscles of your body to move and do work. Physical activity is everything you do during the day that requires your body to move: walking, cleaning, washing the car, cooking, gardening, or playing active games with children.

The nutrition information in this book and the Healthy Eating Pyramid are summaries of hundreds—possibly thousands—of research findings; they represent the current consensus. In 1990, the best consensus about physical activity and good health resulted from reviewing all the studies that had reported on these issues. At that time the recommendation was that individuals should exercise three to five times a week at 60–90% of their maximum heart rate for 20–60 minutes per session.[2] Some of you may have heard this recommendation before.

Since that time, additional research has been completed. Several studies have shown that physical activity does not have to be completed in one continuous session but could be broken up into exercise bouts, or short 10-minute sessions. For example, participating in three 10-minute exercise sessions provides the same health benefits as participating in one 30-minute exercise session.[3] Short exercise sessions could also reduce the risk of heart disease.[4]

Instead of having to reserve a 30-minute block of time every day, a person could walk briskly for 10 minutes in the morning, take a 10-minute walk at lunch, and work in the garden or mow the grass for 10 minutes in the evening and get all the benefits of physical activity. With this new research in mind, the recommendation for physical activity has been revised to the one you've already seen at least three times in this book: "Every adult should accumulate at least 30 minutes of moderate-intensity physical activity on most, preferably all, days of the week."[5]

This recommendation contains all the information you need to get the most out of your physical activity. When striving to improve cardiovascular endurance, the letters "F.I.T." can help you remember three principles to make your physical activity effective. The letters stand for **F**requency, **I**ntensity, and **T**ime. By carefully rereading the physical activity recommendation above, it is easy to see how each principle is used.

According to the recommendation, you should try to participate in physical activity on most, preferably all, days of the week. This is the *frequency*. The *intensity* of your activity should be moderate, and the minimum amount of accumulated exercise *time* should be around 30 minutes.

What if you cannot exercise every day? If you can't go every day, you can still get the health benefits by exercising three to five times a week, but you may have to exercise for more than 30 minutes. The whole idea is to accumulate activity. Some athletes train four times a week and rest on the off days. However, on the days they do train, they work very hard, and afterward their bodies need rest. The amount of exercise they complete is about the same as someone who exercises every day for less time at a lower intensity.

Intensity is a measure of the amount of work the cardiovascular system is performing or the amount of energy a specific activity requires—for example, when you run, your breathing increases as your body's need for oxygen increases. The intensity of running is high—it requires a lot of energy and oxygen. If you ran really fast for two to three minutes, your heart would start beating as fast as it could. At this level of intensity, you would reach a maximum heart rate, or the most your heart can beat in one minute. This is maximum intensity—100%.

You might be wondering what your maximum heart rate is. It is easy to calculate because it is directly related to your age; gender is not a factor.[6] In Table 10.1, find your age or the age closest to your age. The heart rate (HR) value next to the age is your estimated maximum heart rate. If you ran as hard as you could for a few minutes, the fastest your heart would beat would be close to this number.

Age	Max HR	Age	Max HR	Age	Max HR	Age	Max HR	Age	Max HR
18	195	32	186	46	176	60	166	74	156
20	194	34	184	48	174	62	165	76	155
22	193	36	183	50	173	64	163	78	153
24	191	38	181	52	172	66	162	80	152
26	190	40	180	54	170	68	160	82	151
28	188	42	179	56	169	70	159	84	149
30	187	44	177	58	167	72	158	86	148

The formula to calculate your maximum heart rate = 208 − (0.7 x age).

Table 10.1 Estimated maximum heart rate according to age

For a 50-year-old who is fit and running up a hill, the fastest his or her heart would beat is about 173 beats per minute (see Table 10.1). If this activity were part of a regular lifestyle habit, this person would be considered very fit and would receive all the benefits associated with physical activity. But let's be realistic; there are only a fraction of 50-year-olds who actually like to run up big hills on a regular basis.

When you exercise at your maximum heart rate, you expend a lot of energy and cause your body to strain to keep going. This level of intensity is required for some sports—playing a vigorous game of basketball requires this kind of intensity, for example. For those who are fit, this level of intensity is normal and can even be enjoyable. But it is not required for good health. In fact, exercising at a high intensity can cause injuries if you are unfit, and the discomfort that sometimes comes with high-intensity activity may discourage you from doing any physical activity. Unless you are already fit, it is not advisable to participate in activities that cause your heart to work at its maximum rate.

How often do you find yourself breathing rapidly when walking? Unless you are pushing a stroller or walking up a hill or hiking in steep terrain, the intensity of walking is generally not too high. How about when you are sleeping? As you can guess, very little work is done during sleep, and the intensity is very low. Moderate-intensity activities are those that make you work hard enough to substantially increase your heart rate but are not intense enough to cause discomfort.

To get the health benefits of regular exercise, it is suggested that your intensity be somewhere between 60% and 90% of your maximum heart rate. This is known as the ideal intensity. For example, if I were 20 years old, my estimated maximum heart rate would be 194 beats per minute (see Table 10.1), and 60% to 90% of 194 is 116 to 175 beats per minute, or the ideal intensity. If you are exercising and your heart rate is at the ideal intensity, which means the intensity is neither too high nor too low, it still gives you benefits.

How do you find your heart rate? You can measure your pulse by placing your fingers on the carotid artery at the front of your neck or on the artery in your wrist (count how many times your heart beats in one minute), or you can wear a heart-rate monitor. These methods allow you to measure how fast your heart is beating, but if you are preoccupied with measuring your heart rate, you may not be having much fun. There is a better way to assess your intensity, and it's a lot easier. It's called the Talk Test.

The Talk Test

The Talk Test is an easy guide to help you determine the appropriate exercise intensity. If you can talk without too much difficulty while you are exercising, you are most likely in your ideal intensity range. If you are really breathing hard and you can barely talk, you are probably working at a very high intensity. If you can quote extensive poetry without pausing for a breath, you probably need to step it up a little. Remember, don't get caught up in trying to determine your exact exercise heart rate and intensity every time you exercise. If you are playing basketball or jogging, don't worry about your intensity—just enjoy yourself. The most important thing is to exercise often and have fun doing activities you enjoy.

Most physical activities that cause you to work in the ideal intensity range are considered moderate-intensity activities. Figure 10.1 shows a list of common activities that are moderate in intensity; there are quite a few, as you can see. Those listed at the top are more vigorous and those on the bottom are less vigorous. To get the recommended amount of physical activity, spend more time doing less vigorous activities and less time doing intense activities. All the activities in Figure 10.1 promote good health. It is not a complete list; there are hundreds of other activities you may like that are not included. Pick activities you like to do and, if you wonder if your intensity is sufficient, use the Talk Test to check.

Low-intensity to moderate-intensity activities, when done for as little as 30 minutes a day, provide benefits. Low- to moderate-intensity activities include pleasure walking, climbing stairs, gardening, yard work, moderate to heavy housework, dancing, and home exercise. More vigorous aerobic activities, such as brisk walking, running, swimming, bicycling,

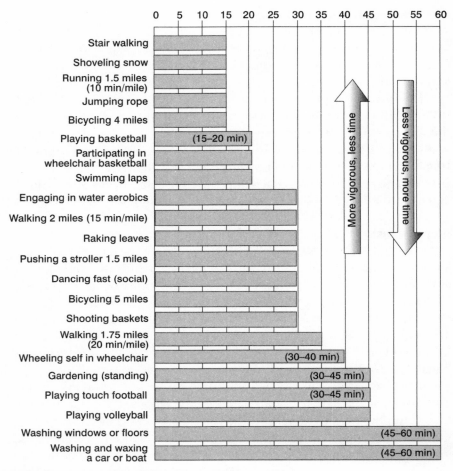

Figure 10.1 Moderate-intensity physical activities
(from www.cdc.gov/nccdphp/dnpa/physical/recommendations/adults.htm)

rollerblading, and jumping rope, done three or four times a week for 30 to 60 minutes are best for improving the fitness of the heart and lungs and provide additional health benefits.

A Few Things to Remember

Perhaps you have heard the saying, "No pain, no gain." It refers to the belief that unless you experience some pain while exercising, you won't gain any benefit. All the benefits of physical activity are available without the presence of pain. Some pain (such as that associated with a sprained ankle or major medical procedure) requires you to stop all exercise until your body heals, and everyone experiences the occasional aches and pains of everyday life. But if you experience pain while exercising, stop doing that type of exercise or reduce the intensity; any pain beyond daily bumps and bruises is not a requirement for being physically active.

A concept closely related to this notion of pain and gain is the overload principle. This principle is based on the fact that in order for a muscle or the cardiovascular system to become stronger and more efficient, it has to be subjected to loads greater than those to which it is accustomed. This is true for almost everything in life. If you want to become a better public speaker, you have to practice speaking in public. If you want to become fit, you have to put your body into situations where fitness can be developed.

According to the overload principle, increases in fitness are possible only when you make your body do physical activities at a greater intensity than usual. Most young adults won't improve their level of fitness by walking. Young adults need more intense activity to get the same benefits an adult gets with less intense activity. Young adults could improve their fitness by hiking, biking, walking up hills, or jogging. Brisk walking is the most common form of physical activity for older adults to improve fitness.

You have to overload the system with slightly more difficult activities than you usually perform, but don't bite off more than you can chew. A popular way many people use to "start slowly" is to enter a weekend softball tournament. A day or two after spending an entire day sprinting around bases, some people experience severe muscle soreness. The intensity of a softball game is greater than what they usually do. If your intensity progresses too quickly, you will likely get sore. It is no fun, and soreness doesn't have to be part of your healthy lifestyle.

Increases in physical activity are best attained with gradual increases in workload. If you are currently sedentary or if you took the 1.5-mile fitness test in chapter 9 and determined that you have a low fitness level, you should start with short bouts of low-intensity activity. For example, take 10 minutes and walk around the block. Gradually increase the number and/or length of bouts until you can accumulate 30 minutes of moderately intense activity. Don't increase the frequency, intensity, or duration of your activity until you are comfortable working at your current level. As you gradually adjust to physical activity, your body also changes gradually, and you don't get sore.

Another important concept to remember is the idea of reversibility or "use it or lose it." Once you begin participating in regular physical activity, your health will improve and your fitness will increase. However, these improvements quickly reverse if you don't maintain the physical activity. The beneficial physiological changes that occur with regular endurance activities revert to their previous state, and if you don't use your newfound fitness, your body reverts to its previous condition—your lowest level of fitness. The only way to keep the body fit is to continually subject it to physical activity that keeps the body in a higher state of fitness and health.

There are two ways we lose fitness. One happens as we age, and the other happens when we stop being physically active. As we age, our ability to do physical work declines. After about age 25–30, we lose about 10% of our fitness every decade.[7,8] It doesn't matter if we are sedentary or extremely fit, the decline appears to be related to the aging process; it's a part of life. For most Americans, the age-related decline in fitness is more

---

All the benefits of physical activity are available without the presence of pain.

---

pronounced because of the decrease in physical activity. Furthermore, between the ages of 20 and 30, physical activity participation drops dramatically for most people. This covers the single largest decline in fitness that occurs during a typical life, and it is not age related; it is caused by a reduction in physical activity.

To demonstrate how rapidly this reduction can occur, researchers recruited 20-year-old males who consented to be bedridden for three weeks.[9] At the end of the three weeks, their fitness levels had declined by 15%. To really make things interesting, they tracked the men for the next 30 years to see what happened to them. After 30 years, their body fat doubled from 14% to 28%, and their fitness declined by 14%. Three weeks of bed rest in these same men at 20 years of age had a more profound impact on fitness than did three decades of aging.[10]

After 30 years, they called the men together and put them through a six-month fitness program. After the program, their fitness levels improved dramatically, but not quite to the levels they had been at as young men. These studies show that fitness levels are fluid and change rapidly according to lifestyle. Our fitness increases when we are physically active and decreases when we are sedentary.

Sooner or later, everyone fails to maintain regular exercise. When this occurs, the important thing is to start exercising again as soon as you can. When you stop having an active lifestyle, you stop getting the benefits.

The more support you have from others and the more you enjoy your activities, the more likely you will be to stay active and maintain the benefits associated with physical activity.

The last thing to remember when beginning an exercise program is the principle of individuality. Studies of the genetic differences among individuals have shown that changes in fitness differ greatly among individuals.[11] In one study of adults who participated in a 12-week exercise program, there was a very large difference in improvement in fitness levels. Even though the adults started with the same levels of fitness and did the same amount of exercise, certain individuals experienced large increases in fitness, while others experienced only slight increases. These results are primarily the result of genetic differences among individuals.[12]

Some people inherit the ability to sprint fast or jump high, while others inherit high levels of fitness. Even though there are clear genetic differences among individuals, genetics is only part of the picture. Everyone benefits from regular exercise, even if they aren't world-class athletes. It is possible that you may not experience significant increases in fitness even after several months of activity. A notable increase in endurance is only one change that occurs in your body. Other changes happen that aren't as obvious, so don't get discouraged.

Medical Clearance

Don't forget to make sure you have medical clearance before you begin to exercise. Men over age 40 and women over age 50 who plan to begin a new, vigorous physical activity program should consult a physician first to be sure they do not have heart disease or other health problems. If you are not sure if you should see your physician, review the medical clearance questions at the end of chapter 9.

Warm-up and Cool Down

Each time you exercise, you should begin with a short warm-up. Warming up is important because it lets your heart rate increase gradually, rather than jumping suddenly from a low resting heart rate to an elevated heart rate. Warming up also warms the muscles, making them more flexible and preparing them for activity. When you warm up, begin exercising at a low intensity; walking is a good warm-up activity (low intensity, slowly elevates your heart rate). Regardless of the activity you choose, go easy for the first five minutes. When you feel yourself starting to sweat, you are likely warm enough to begin vigorous activity.

After you complete your activity, cool down by continuing to move around for a few minutes; a few minutes of slow walking is a good way to cool down. This keeps the blood circulating around the body. This is also a good time to stretch, while the muscles are still warm.

Choosing Shoes and Exercise Clothing

You'll notice that the list of moderate-intensity activities in Figure 10.1 is missing activities that require specialized or expensive equipment. For example, snow skiing, water skiing, golfing, and backpacking are missing from the list. This was done purposely to demonstrate that a lifestyle of regular physical activity does not require costly equipment or memberships to clubs. When selecting exercise clothing, the same rationale is true—you do not have to have the best looking or most expensive clothes to enjoy physical activity. This also applies to the type of exercise shoes you wear. There is a wide range of prices and styles for exercise shoes. To choose the correct type of shoes, just remember that court-type shoes work best on court surfaces and running shoes work well for running. Everything else is just marketing propaganda. Shoes worn for running or walking should have a thick, cushioned heel. This reduces the amount of impact felt in the feet and legs and helps prevent some joint soreness, especially in the knee. Court shoes are generally designed to support forward, backward, and lateral movements. Generally the soles are sturdier than the soles on running shoes, and they may cover the ankle, which can provide some resistance to ankle sprains. Shop around or wait for shoe sales; with so many stores selling shoes, it is not hard to find good shoes at a reasonable price.

When it is really hot outside, remember these three things about the clothes you should wear: light colors, lightweight, loose fitting. Light-colored clothing reflects some of the sun's rays and lightweight clothing doesn't trap warm air close to your skin. Loose-fitting clothes also allow the warm air to escape. Wear a hat, try to stay in the shade, drink lots of water, and, if you can, avoid exercising outside during the hottest times of the day (between 10:00 a.m. and 6:00 p.m.).

When it's really cold outside, simply remember the opposite about the clothes you wear: dark colors, heavy weight (layers are best), tight fitting. The dark colors actually absorb the sun's rays, and the different layers of clothes trap warm air next to the body (the same principle for tighter fit, too). If you get too hot, you can always take off a layer. As much as 70% of your body heat can be lost from your head and hands; wearing a hat and mittens prevents most of this heat loss and makes you more comfortable; if you get too hot, take them off.

What about Your Muscles?

Have you ever done any of these activities: carried a small child in your arms, carried your luggage while traveling, shoveled snow, carried groceries into your kitchen, helped a friend move furniture, mowed the lawn (with a manual mower, not one that is self-propelled), carried golf clubs for 18 holes, or changed a tire? All these activities are part of our daily lives. All these activities require muscle strength and endurance (an important but usually neglected component of fitness). The ability to do a strenuous activity, like carrying a toddler, is an example of muscle endurance, while lifting a tire into the trunk of a car requires muscle strength.

In Greek mythology the strongest man in the world was Milo. When he was a child, one of the cows in the family herd had a bull calf. Each day Milo would go out to the pasture and lift the calf off the ground. As the calf grew, Milo had to work harder and harder to lift the weight. After many years of lifting, Milo could lift the bull off the ground and carry it on his shoulders all the way around the stadium at Olympia in Greece, an impressive feat. By overloading his muscles every day, his strength increased, and he was able to lift the increasing weight of the bull.

Each pound of muscle uses about 25 calories every day. That may not seem like much, but over a month or year, it adds up. That's why having muscle helps prevent weight gain. Losing muscle makes you more likely to gain weight.

Then there's the story about Mike. Mike played a few sports in high school and college, but when he graduated, he took a desk job. Every day Mike slaved away at his computer and shuffled paper. Each day, the muscles in his arms and legs slowly weakened and mostly disappeared. One hot summer day, the water bottle on top of the water cooler ran dry. Like Milo lifting the bull, he lifted a full bottle of water (about 40 pounds) onto his shoulder. Instead of heroically carrying it across the room and placing it into position, he strained under the weight and collapsed to the floor, a very embarrassing feat. The "use it or lose it" principle was confirmed in Mike's case.

Mike's sedentary lifestyle and job contributed to his muscle weakness. He had difficulty carrying his luggage or shoveling snow and dirt, and he tired quickly when he tried to carry his toddler. He lost muscle strength, muscle endurance, and many other health and quality-of-life benefits. Contrary to what you may have heard, his muscles did not turn to fat. It is impossible for muscle to be replaced with fat. His muscles simply got smaller and weaker, and he gained weight in obvious places—around his stomach, hips, and thighs.

The loss of muscle not only reduced his strength, but it also reduced the number of calories his body burned throughout the day. Muscle is a contractile tissue that requires energy 24 hours a day just to exist. Forty-five percent of the body weight of an adult is muscle mass; the typical adult has about 50–70 pounds of muscle.[13] Each pound of muscle uses about 25 calories every day. That may not seem like much, but over a month or year, it adds up. That's why having muscle helps prevent weight gain. Losing muscle makes you more likely to gain weight. It also makes you less able to perform basic physical functions when you become elderly.

Since fitness declines with age, researchers originally speculated that muscle strength might also decline with age, but this is not true. After age 20, most adults lose about one half pound of muscle every year. At age 65, most will have lost 25% of their peak muscle strength. But unlike fitness, loss of muscle comes from disuse, not the aging process.[14,15] Studies have shown that men in their 60s and 70s who strength train regularly have muscles that look and perform as well as those of inactive men in their 20s and 30s.[16] Just getting older doesn't mean you have to give up muscle strength and the benefits of being strong.

How Much?

Besides regular physical activity, the consensus of scientific opinion suggests that all adults should do some strength training at least twice a week.[17,18] Only 11% of adults age 65 and older strength train two or more days a week. The highest percent of the population that lifts weights is young adults.

To get the benefits of strength training, you should work all the major muscle groups in your body, including your arms, chest, shoulders, abdomen, back, and legs. Repeat each exercise 10–15 times. If you have access to a weight room, you should have no trouble keeping your muscles strong, but weight-lifting equipment is not required. All you have to do to keep your muscles strong is work against resistance; sit-ups and push-ups are great exercises. Free weights, barbells, resistance bands, and even exercising in water can also provide good resistance. You can maintain leg strength by doing any type of exercise that requires you to use your legs (jogging, aerobics, climbing stairs, bicycling, yoga, and walking). If your regular physical activity consists mostly of activities that strengthen the legs, try to do some strength training for your upper body by adding push-ups and sit-ups to your activity during the week.

Don't expect your muscles to change overnight. Just like the benefits of physical activity, the benefits of strength training take time. Most people start to experience improvements in strength after six weeks. It is common to experience a 20–40% increase in strength after several months. If you plan to go to a gym with weight-training equipment, ask the trainers for assistance with the machines. And go easy the first time.

Use the guesstimate method to determine how much weight to use for each lift. Guess a weight you think you can lift 10 times and try it. If you can't do eight lifts in a row, the weight is too heavy; try a lighter one. If you can lift the weight more than 15 times in a row, the weight is probably too light; chose a slightly heavier weight. If you struggle just a bit to finish 10 lifts at the weight you choose, you are using the right weight. After lifting for several days, you'll find you can lift the same weight more easily.

What about someone who has a job that requires heavy lifting or vigorous physical labor? If you have that type of job, such as working construction or caring for the elderly, you probably don't need to worry about strength training because you already do it. The amount of work your muscles do every day on the job enables you to maintain your muscle strength.

Strength training program at home

The Centers for Disease Control and Prevention has produced a nice online program to get you started on a simple 12-week strength training program you can do in your own home. You can find this program at:

www.cdc.gov/nccdphp/dnpa/physical/growing_stronger/exercises/index.htm

If you want more information on strength training, visit your local YMCA or fitness center, or try reading Susie Dinan's *Strength Training for Beginners*, HarperCollins Publishers, 2003.

POINTS TO REMEMBER

- When you exercise, you get the benefits; when you stop exercising, the benefits stop.

- Accumulate at least 30 minutes of moderate-intensity physical activity on most, preferably all, days of the week.

- The Talk Test is an easy method for maintaining proper exercise intensity.

- "No pain, no gain" is a myth.

- Strength training is great exercise and can improve your quality of life.

PART THREE

How

SUSTAINED EFFORT ▶

MOTIVATION ▶

PROGRESS ▶

CHANGE ▶

CONFIDENCE ▶

SOCIAL SUPPORT ▶

REALISTIC GOALS ▶

ENVIRONMENT ▶

COMMUNITY ▶

PARTNER ▶

HEALTH-PROMOTION PROGRAM ▶

Being Physically Active for Life

Respect your efforts, respect yourself.
Self-respect leads to self-discipline; when you
have both firmly under your belt, that's real power.
—Clint Eastwood (1930–)

IN THE FIRST SECTION OF THIS BOOK WE DISCUSSED WHY a healthy lifestyle is important. The last few chapters have shown you what comprises a healthy lifestyle. You now have all the information you need to understand the health benefits available to you when you choose a healthy lifestyle. Now we have arrived at a critical juncture. All the information about good health and quality of life is of no value unless it can motivate and inspire you to change, and until you change your diet and become physically active—two very difficult behaviors to alter—the benefits we've discussed will elude you. It all comes down to this; this is where the rubber meets the road. I wrote this book to help you learn why a healthy lifestyle is important and to give you the tools, tips, and plans to incorporate what you have learned into your life.

I have devoted my professional life to helping people adopt healthy lifestyles. If I've learned one thing in my efforts, it is that many people struggle to eat a healthy diet and even more people struggle to stay physically active. The struggle comes not because people don't care—almost everyone cares about their health, body weight, and quality of life. The struggle to adopt and maintain a healthy lifestyle is caused by a combination of personal reasons, the environment in which we live, and a lack of community resources. All of these together either support or hinder our efforts. I'm sure that you have experienced this struggle firsthand.

Think of a behavior you have tried to change (think of any of New Year's resolutions you may have made in the past). Maybe you tried to lose weight, reduce your stress, eat better, get more sleep, get out of debt, spend more time with family, or find a new job. We all know how the process works. It starts when you reach the point where you are no longer happy with your life. You gather enough determination to do something about it. You might set some goals, talk with friends or family, put together a plan, and begin.

Your initial efforts are sustained by the reservoir of determination you built before you started. Slowly, ever so slowly, that reservoir drains as you experience setbacks, disappointments, or roadblocks in your plans to make the new behavior permanent. Your motivation stays high when you start to see progress and experience some of the benefits of the changes you have made. But without evidence of progress, your reservoir may drain completely; your resolve might weaken or you might revert back to the way you were.

As hard as it is to make permanent changes, many people are able to do it. People have quit smoking, some have lost weight and kept it off, and others have gotten out of debt. We know change is possible. Even though most people don't get adequate exercise and eat right, about 25% of the population does. How do they do it when so many others fail?

Let's take a closer look at the reasons why you failed to make the desired change in your behavior. Check your reasons against the list of reasons below. Put a check mark next to the ones that contributed to your failure. (There may be other reasons not on this list; include those in the "Other" category.)

___ I gave up during an especially stressful or busy time.

___ My family and friends did not provide much support.

___ I lost confidence in my ability to keep it up.

___ I didn't see any of the benefits I thought would come with the new behavior.

___ I failed to reach my goal.

___ I lost my motivation.

___ My environment did not support my new behavior.

___ My community did not support me in maintaining my new behavior.

___ I was doing well, but the temptation was too great and I went back to my old ways.

_____ It was a lot of hard work, and it just wasn't worth it.

_____ Other_____

Many dedicated researchers are trying to figure out what it takes for people to successfully change behaviors. These experts have identified a number of traits common among people who adopt and maintain new behaviors for a long time[1-3]; the "reasons for failure" list was derived from this research. The main reasons for failure often include lack of confidence, lack of social support, failure to understand the pros and cons of a new behavior, failure to set realistic goals, and poor support from the environment or community.

The researchers found that the opposite is also true. Those who make successful long-term behavior changes have confidence in their ability to maintain the new behavior and they receive support from friends, family, and coworkers. They also value the benefits of the new behavior more than the benefits of the old behavior. They set realistic goals, and they live in homes and work at places with supportive environments.

Prevention of chronic diseases, extension of life, and improvement of quality of life are all possible benefits of healthy behaviors. To help you be physically active for life, let's stack the deck in your favor by talking about how to avoid failure.

Support from Others

It's tough to go it alone. Whether you are already physically active or you're trying to become active, help from others makes it easier. When you include others in your exercise, you gain many advantages. Suppose you walk briskly every morning. One day you wake up and the temperature has fallen and it feels cold. If you know your walking partner is waiting for you at the corner, you can't bail out on her. It's just not nice to leave your friends out in the cold, wondering if you are coming. This social pressure to be nice to your partner may be enough to cause you to grab your coat and get walking. If you know someone is depending on you, you are more likely to participate.

 INSIDE THE ALDANA HOME ▶▶▶ *Exercising with others is a social experience. I don't know if it counts as a real date, but each day I spend a little time exercising with my wife. It's a great time for us to communicate, plan, and be together. When one of us doesn't feel like going, a pouting face and a sincere "pleeeeease" can almost always get us out the door together. As we walk or jog, we see other groups walking. A neighbor*

who is blind walks with the aid of a friend. We see whole groups of women walking in the early morning hours. We also see young mothers pushing children in strollers. The kids love the ride, and mom is getting a good workout.

There are many ways others can encourage you to be physically active.[4] They can give you a ride to the gym, tell you about a fun run, or talk to you about the benefits of exercise. It's encouraging when someone asks how you are doing with your exercise habit; it is a way for them to show you they really care. One married woman tells her husband how much she loves him and how much she wants to spend many years together with him. This emotional support is enough to get him exercising.

It is not too bold to buy a spouse a treadmill as a birthday gift. Some may think it is an awful gift because it may carry the unspoken message, "I think you are overweight and out of shape." The true message that accompanies a gift like this should be (whether spoken or written), "I love you and I want to be with you for a long time."

One of the best forms of support is giving and receiving positive feedback and encouragement. It means a lot when someone notices your improved appearance and says, "Wow, you look great!"

INSIDE THE ALDANA HOME ▸▸▸ *I recall seeing a husband drop off his wife near the door of a church and then drive off to park the car before walking in to join her. I was impressed that he was such a gentleman, but I wondered if he really understood the benefits of physical activity. His wife was middle-aged, sedentary, and obese. I never said anything, but in my mind I thought, "If this gentleman really loved his wife, he would tell her so and encourage her to walk across the parking lot with him." Better yet, they both could have easily left the car home and walked to the church. He could have been supportive of her being physically active and still been the perfect gentleman.*

Boyfriends, girlfriends, neighbors, children, and even pets make great exercise partners. Tell your friends and family that you are serious about getting adequate physical activity and you want their support. Even if they don't support you, deep down I think they will be silently envious and wishing they had your commitment to being physically active.

Pros and Cons of Physical Activity

Below are two lists. One is a list of exercise benefits, and the other is a list of exercise barriers or dislikes. Check the benefits that are important to you; then check the negative aspects that match your attitude toward exercise. Don't hide your true thoughts and feelings; if some aspect of physical activity really bothers you, check it.

Benefits of exercise I like	Effects of exercise I dislike and barriers that keep me from being active
___I have more energy.	___I don't like to get sweaty.
___I like the way it makes me look.	___I don't have time.
___I'm able to maintain a healthy weight.	___I don't have any money.
___It reduces my stress.	___The weather is bad.
___I sleep better.	___I live in an unsafe neighborhood.
___It helps prevent chronic disease.	___There are no parks, sidewalks, or bicycle paths near my home.
___It helps keep my cholesterol low.	___It's hard to get into the mood.
___It improves my self-confidence.	___I'm lazy.
___I spend time with friends and family.	___Exercise is painful.
___It gives me a chance to get outside.	___I don't like sports.
___It prevents osteoporosis.	___I'm embarrassed to be seen exercising.
___It is fun.	___No one will exercise with me.
	___I don't have exercise clothes, shoes, or equipment.
	___I need to watch my children.
	___I'm pregnant or nursing.
	___I have an illness or injury that makes it difficult or painful to be active.

To achieve your goal of being active for life, the benefits you checked on the left need to be more important than the barriers and dislikes you checked on the right. If the two are equally important, you are more likely to stop being physically active. If the barriers are greater and more numerous than the benefits, you are less likely to be physically active and are therefore less likely to get the benefits. Your success can be determined by how you perceive these benefits and barriers.[5] Here are some ideas to help you overcome the barriers you might face. Refer to these ideas when you are looking for an excuse not to exercise.

"I don't have time to exercise."

Lack of time is the most common exercise barrier. To help you find 30 minutes in your day complete the following activity:

There are activities that you must do every day and there are activities you want to do every day. I have listed the most common activities in the table below. In the rows that are blank, write in any daily activities you do that are not already listed. Now for the hard part: write down how much time you spend each day next to each activity. There are only 24 hours in a day so your total hours cannot exceed 24. Use a pencil because most people have to erase and adjust times to make the total hours add up to 24 hours. I've put the time allotment of a typical adult in the last column to help guide you.

Activities you *must* do every day	Time you spend each day in each activity	Typical adult
sleep		8 hrs
work, including housework		8 hrs
bathe, get dressed		1 hr
eat		1.5 hr
commute/travel		1 hr
spend time with loved ones		.5 hr
exercise		0 hr
Activities you *want to* do every day		
watch TV		2 hr
visit with friends or family after work		.5 hr
enjoy a hobby		.5 hr
do things on the computer		.5 hr
read		.5 hr
TOTAL	24 hours	24 hours

Now that you have an idea of what your average day looks like, there are two ways to find time to exercise. You can combine it with activities you must do or want to do, or you can make exercise a priority and make room for it on your "must do" list. Really busy people combine exercise with the other activities of the day. For example, if you have to go to work, park your car further away from your destination and walk; use stairs instead of the elevator; go for a walk during your lunch break. Think of household chores as opportunities to exercise. Sweeping, cleaning windows, washing cars, or gardening can all be good sources of exercise. Mow the yard with a push mower. When you are spending time with loved ones, make physical activity part of your time together. Why not go for a walk together or play a sport? Start a hobby that requires physical activity, such as golf or gardening.

To make exercise a priority, you will need to spend less time doing one of your daily activities. The average American spends two hours watching TV every day. Watch 30 minutes less TV and you've got time to go for a walk.

"I lack motivation."
- Motivation comes when you are convinced that the effort required to exercise is worth the benefits received.
- If being lazy means being too tired to get up and exercise, then exercise is just what you need. Expending energy in physical activity can actually make you more energetic and productive. As your cardiovascular system becomes more efficient, you have more energy throughout the day.
- If you still lack motivation to exercise, reread chapter 9 and see what benefits you will be missing by remaining sedentary.

"I have poor health."
- Generally, when you are sick or ill, you should avoid strenuous exercise until you are recovered. Some physicians suggest there is no harm in exercising when you have a cold, but it is not safe to exercise when you have the flu.
- Walking is always a safe, effective choice of exercise, regardless of your illness or injury—unless you have a specific recommendation from your physician not to engage in regular exercise.
- If you have a specific injury, try activities that use the other parts of your body. For example, if your legs are injured, try swimming or lifting weights—these activities are often therapeutic to the injury because of increased breathing and blood circulation.
- Ultimately, you are the best judge of whether or not you should exercise. If you have concerns, talk to your physician.

"It hurts when I exercise."
- You may experience temporary or even chronic pain when exercising (running or jogging can be painful for some individuals, usually from differences in hip and knee stability or from past injuries). If you have pain every time you do a certain activity, try something else.
- Try walking, riding a bicycle, swimming, or using exercise equipment designed to reduce joint impact.
- Sometimes you may experience pain because the intensity of the activity you are doing is too high; lower the intensity.

"I'm self-conscious when others see me exercise."
- Try to exercise with friends or relatives who are supportive and who are at about the same level of fitness.
- Exercise in the privacy of your own home.
- Exercise early in the morning or late in the evening. If you choose to exercise outside while it is dark, never go alone.

"The weather is too bad."
- Exercise during the more comfortable hours of the day. Instead of exercising in the heat of the day, go out in the morning or evening.
- If it is too hot or too cold to be outside, exercise inside. Many malls open their doors early to allow walking inside, and many gyms and fitness centers have extended hours or are open 24 hours a day.
- Dress appropriately for the weather.

"I don't have access to exercise facilities or equipment."
- Some of the best exercise is free and requires no equipment. (Refer to the list of suggested activities in Figure 10.1.)
- You don't have to participate in sports, which often require specialized equipment.
- Many places of employment provide exercise facilities, but if your employer does not provide on-site exercise facilities, see if they have or can obtain discounts to local fitness or recreation centers.

"I don't like to get sweaty."
- Exercise in the morning before it gets too hot.
- Exercise in a gym or other air-conditioned building.
- Walk or jog on a treadmill with a fan blowing on you.
- Swim.

"I live in an unsafe neighborhood."
- Never exercise outside alone; always take a partner.
- Never exercise outside after dark.
- Mornings and lunchtime are a lot safer than evenings.
- Check with your employer to see if there are safe places where you can exercise while you are at work.
- If all else fails, exercise at home with videos or by doing housework.

"There are no parks, sidewalks, or bicycle paths near my home."
- Build an exercise-friendly community with grassroots efforts at the city level.
- Check with your city to see who might already be making efforts to build trails and pathways and offer your help and support. Many communities have done a great job making their streets exercise friendly, thanks to community support.
- Try to find relatively safe places to walk, play, or ride.

"No one will exercise with me."
- Check with your local YMCA or community center about walking groups in your area.
- Post flyers around popular walking areas to invite people to form a walking or exercise group.
- Watch for people who are exercising outside at the same time of day you exercise. Be friendly, stop and walk with one of them, and you'll have an exercise partner before you know it.

"I need to watch my children."
- Newborns can be safely tucked into a stroller and pushed around the block.
- Children love to ride bicycles; go on a bike ride together or have your child ride while you walk.
- Chasing children and cleaning offer plenty of physical activity in themselves!
- Mow the yard or wash the car while watching your children play.
- You have to mop the floor more often when you have children, so don't call it mopping, call it exercising.

"I'm pregnant or nursing."
- If you were physically active when you became pregnant, there are rarely any reasons why you cannot continue your activity during pregnancy.
- Check with your physician about refraining from vigorous activity.
- Infants don't nurse all day. There are plenty of 30-minute blocks of time when you can get a break from the demands of motherhood. Let a trusted adult tend your child or take your child with you and go for a walk. Do it for your sanity and your health.

Other Stick-to-It Strategies

In the past decade, manufacturers have developed small electronic and mechanical step counters. These little devices, which are about the size of a pack of matches and clip to your belt or the waistband of your clothes, automatically keep track of every step you take. Many people wear them every day. They act as a constant reminder that you need to move to be physically active. A good level of physical activity for one day has been defined as taking ten thousand steps. Inexpensive pedometers are available at sporting good stores or from online stores such as www.pedometer.com and www.pedometerusa.com.

Use reminders. You will be more likely to go for a walk during your lunch break if you have your walking shoes with you. A reminder could be as simple as taking your exercise clothes out the night before so you can find them easily in the morning, get dressed, and get out the door. Dogs are excellent reminders. They know when you skip a day or forget to take them out. I suppose dogs have some instinctive desire to be outside going for a walks, because they love it. For dogs, a walk may be the only exciting thing they get to do all day.

One of the best ways to increase your chances of staying active is to find something you enjoy. No one likes to do something they do not enjoy. If your exercise or physical activity is something you don't particularly like, it's not likely to be a regular part of your life. Experiment with different activities. Brisk walking is the most common activity for adults,[6,7] but if you don't like to walk, don't. Try swimming, bicycling, hiking, rollerblading, or even golf (without a cart) instead. Gardening is another great activity. There is something for everyone; the number of different physical activities you can do is practically endless.

Exercise Confidence

Researchers have known for some time that one of the best predictors of regular physical activity is a person's confidence in his or her ability to be active.[8,9] People who are confident in their ability to be active make time to exercise and seem to maintain their activity over the long term.[10]

You can rate your own level of confidence. On a scale of 1–5 (1 being the lowest and 5 the highest), how would you describe your confidence in your ability to be regularly physically active for life?

Low confidence				High confidence
1	2	3	4	5

If your level is a 1 or 2—Do you know why you don't feel more confident? Which of the barriers listed previously in this chapter is keeping you from being confident? Can you think of ways to overcome those barriers?

If your level is a 3—You are halfway there; the number of barriers you perceive is about equal to the number of benefits you believe you will receive. You may feel inadequate because you have been sedentary for a long time, but think about the benefits you can get by being active. You didn't suddenly become unfit; it took some time. Likewise, don't expect to improve your fitness overnight. If you start slowly and stay physically active for at least six weeks, you should start to see changes. Most importantly, have fun being active; as you do this, your confidence will increase.

If your level is a 4 or 5—You are probably active now. The key is to maintain your activity level. Be ready to overcome lapses. Stress, work pressure, family trials, or major life changes have a tendency to derail your daily patterns and cause you to stop exercising. Occasional stoppages are no big deal, but failing to get back into your routine of regular physical activity will keep you from enjoying the benefits. It takes discipline to stick to your active lifestyle, but you can do it; lots of other people already have.

Setting Goals

Reaching a goal results in a sense of mastery and achievement. This builds self-esteem and self-confidence, both of which are needed when adopting new behaviors. Individuals who adopt and maintain a lifestyle of physical activity almost always start with a goal. The U.S. Department of Health and Human Services recently became acutely aware of the need to help Americans adopt healthy behaviors and prevent chronic diseases. It now funds large, community-based studies designed to improve nutrition and physical activity levels. It also started the nationwide HealthierUS Initiative, which is described at www.HealthierUS.gov. The purpose of this initiative is to help Americans get good nutrition and participate in regular physical activity. Part of the initiative includes simple steps for improving physical activity. These steps come in the form of small daily goals. The list provided by the HealthierUS Initiative is included below. Select a few simple steps you can do today.

Small Steps to Help You Increase Your Physical Activity
   Walk to work.
   Do sit-ups in front of the TV.
   Walk during lunch hour.
   Walk instead of drive whenever you can.
   Take a family walk after dinner.
   Skate to work instead of drive.
   Mow lawn with push mower.
   Walk to your place of worship instead of drive.
   Walk kids to school.
   Get a dog and walk it.
   Join an exercise group.
   Replace Sunday drive with Sunday walk.
   Do yard work.
   Get off the bus or train one stop early and walk.
   Work around the house.
   Bicycle to the store instead of drive.
   Go for a half-hour walk instead of watching TV.
   Fetch the newspaper yourself.
   Sit up straight at work.
   Wash the car by hand.
   Run when running errands.
   Pace the sidelines at kids' athletic games.
   Take wheels off luggage.
   Choose an activity that fits into your daily life.
   Park farther from the store and walk.
   Ask a friend to exercise with you.
   Exercise with a video if the weather is bad.
   Bike to the barbershop or beauty salon instead of drive.
   If you find it difficult to be active after work, try it before work.
   Take a walk or do desk exercises instead of a cigarette or coffee break.

Perform gardening or home repair activities.

Avoid laborsaving devices.

Take small trips on foot to get your body moving.

Play with your kids 30 minutes a day.

Dance to music.

Keep a pair of comfortable walking or running shoes in your car
and office.

Make a Saturday morning walk a group habit.

Walk briskly in the mall.

Choose activities you enjoy and you'll be more likely to stick with them.

Stretch before bed to give you more energy when you wake.

Take the long way to the water cooler.

Explore new physical activities.

Vary your activities for interest and to broaden the range of benefits.

Take the stairs instead of the escalator.

Swim with your kids.

Walk instead of sitting around.

Take your dog on longer walks.

Walk the beach instead of sunbathing.

Walk to a coworker's desk instead of e-mailing or calling them.

Carry your groceries instead of pushing a cart.

Use a snow shovel instead of a snow blower.

In the future, when your confidence to be physically active starts to wane, read the list again and pick other small steps to try.

For those who are ready to get serious about being physically active, a more aggressive goal may be appropriate. Choose several activities you would like to do regularly. Use the list of small steps above, refer to the list of the moderate physical activities in Figure 10.1 in the last chapter, or pick some other activity. If your fitness level is currently low or if you are sedentary, choose low- to moderate-intensity activities.

Use the following table to fill in your activity plan for a full week. In the activity column, write in the activities you plan to do next to the days you want to do them. Beside each activity, record the amount of time you will spend doing it. As you fill out your schedule, remember the exercise recommendation: *"Every adult should accumulate 30 minutes or more of moderate-intensity physical activity on most, preferably all, days of the week and even more activity is better."* It is okay to make changes to your program; in fact, it is encouraged.

Days	Activity	Duration (minutes)
Monday		
Tuesday		
Wednesday		
Thursday		
Friday		
Saturday		
Sunday		

Try to keep this schedule for the next 12 weeks. To help you keep track of your activity, mark the days you exercise on a calendar or keep a journal. To demonstrate how committed you are, share this goal with a friend or significant other and sign it. Let them know you want their support and ask them to sign it as a witness of your commitment. (Once they've signed it, ask them to exercise with you!)

Signature:_____ Date: _____

Witness:_____ Date: _____

Reward Yourself

If you successfully make small steps to improve your activity or if you reach your physical activity goal, consider giving yourself a reward. This reward should be something to encourage your good behavior. You might consider buying a new pair of exercise shoes or a new outfit. Buy a pedometer to track your activity. Other rewards might include a water bottle, a night out, a massage, a new book, or a small party with friends. A dozen Krispy Kreme doughnuts might not be the best choice.

INSIDE THE ALDANA HOME ►►► *I work approximately 11 miles from my home. I'd love to ride my bicycle to work, but the only route is along a four-lane highway with six inches of space on the edge of the road. I have ridden my bike to work before, but I found it to be a harrowing experience to have cars whizzing by me at 60 miles an hour. At times, the cars' mirrors were only inches away from me. If there were a designated bike path or trail, I and hundreds of others would ride to work every day.*

Like many places, the environment I live in does not support an active lifestyle. Many locations do not have sidewalks or pedestrian crosswalks, and even though pedestrians are supposed to have the right-of-way, anyone who walks a lot will tell you that cars really own the roads. Most suburbs are designed to serve commuters who have automobiles. Anyone who wishes to walk, run, bike, or rollerblade in these areas has to carefully pick routes that are safe from traffic and crime.

A Supportive Environment

Laborsaving devices are another part of the environment we have created that reduce the physical activity we could be getting. These devices include such things as escalators, elevators, cars, drive-through windows at restaurants, golf carts, and snowblowers.

One of the most troubling environmental barriers to appear in the past few years is the discontinuance of recess in elementary schools. Some estimate that 40% of school districts have either eliminated recess or are discussing removing it; many school districts in Texas have already eliminated recess from the daily schedule. In these districts, students are expected to stay inside and have lunch, play quiet games, or study.

All the information about good health
and quality of life is of no value unless it can motivate
and inspire you to change.

The reasons behind the elimination of recess include the perceived lack of time needed to cover more important topics and the observation that students get too excited at recess and use valuable class time to settle down afterwards. This is one of the worst health policies to be enacted in quite some time. It's not surprising that Texas school children have some of the highest obesity rates in the country.[11] Other factors obviously contribute to obesity, but eliminating recess certainly isn't making kids healthier.

Each day most Americans spend one third of the day sleeping, one third working, and one third doing other activities. Many worksites have health-promotion programs for their employees. These programs provide opportunities to exercise, eat healthy foods, and participate in health-promoting activities. If you work outside the home, ask your boss if there is a health-promotion program at your office; if one does not exist, encourage your management to start one. Many worksites that have such programs report that not only are employees healthier, but the company also benefits by having employees who are absent less often, who are more productive, and who have fewer health care expenses.

While at work you might have opportunities to participate in department exercise competitions or company physical activity goals. For example, the employees at the Washoe County School District in Reno, Nevada, enjoy simple, four- to eight-week programs throughout the year that reinforce physical activity and proper nutrition. Programs like this provide the catalyst needed to drive a cultural shift towards health and well-being. These employees get incentives for being active and seem to love the camaraderie. Each day at work, coworkers and administrators support their efforts to be active. They have a very healthy work environment. You can view reports of their success at www.washoe.k12.nv.us/wellness.

Over 60,000 people have participated in California's online work-site physical activity program called Take Action. It was started by the California State Department of Health Services to help working adults stay physically active. You can read more about this program at www.ca-takeaction.com. Another place to get great tips on creating a healthy work environment is at the Web site of the Wellness Councils of America (www.welcoa.org). Long-term physical activity participation is easier with a helpful and supportive environment.

POINTS TO REMEMBER

- Failure is part of the process of making healthy behavioral changes; don't give up if you experience setbacks or failures.

- You can't be regularly physically active without help from others. Identify others who can be active with you.

- Focus on the benefits of exercise you enjoy.

- Evaluate ways you can overcome your exercise barriers.

- Get a pedometer.

- Don't move on to the next chapter until you have set an exercise goal for yourself.

CHAPTER

Healthy Eating for Life

Any change, even a change for the better,
is always accompanied by drawbacks and discomforts.
—Arnold Bennett

I F SCIENTIFIC EVIDENCE COULD GUARANTEE that eating a healthy diet would make you live an additional 50 years without any diseases, there would still be people who wouldn't do it. Health benefits from good nutrition and exercise are wonderful for those who care. For those who really don't care about their health, all the health benefits in the world won't convince them to eat more healthy foods. Food is an interesting part of our existence, it is a paradox. If you don't eat, you will die prematurely; if you eat too much of the wrong kinds of foods, you will die prematurely; and if you eat healthy foods you will most likely live a long, high-quality life.

Most Americans choose to eat too many unhealthy foods. It's the most popular of the three choices because many unhealthy foods are tasty, inexpensive, and convenient. Taste, cost, and convenience are the main reasons many people struggle to eat good foods.[1]

Think about the last meal you ate before you started reading this chapter. List the foods in your mind. Why did you choose those particular foods? Did you decide to eat these foods because of the taste, cost, ease (convenience) of preparation, and nutrition, or was it because you are concerned about your weight? Most likely the foods you eat are determined by one of these factors. Attempts to make improvements in your diet will be more successful if the healthy foods you eat are tasty, affordable, and easy to prepare.

The odds of a person eating more healthy foods are directly related to how ready he or she is to change eating habits.[2] Most Americans want to make changes; 25–60% are already trying to eat healthier.[3]

Which of these statements describes you?
- I already eat a healthy diet.
- Some of the foods I eat are healthy, and I'm willing to try other things to improve my diet.
- I'm not sure I really want to change my diet; I like the way I eat.
- I don't care what I eat.

These statements represent categories that describe how ready people are to make nutrition changes.[4] The categories include those who are currently eating a good diet, those who are exploring the idea of eating better, those who are reluctant, and those who are not concerned about the foods they eat. Everyone fits into one of these groups. Not surprisingly, those who successfully change their eating habits are more likely to explore the idea of eating better, while those who are reluctant or unconcerned might struggle to make good nutrition a part of their lives.

The discussion of I-don't-care-itis in chapter 3 is directed at those who are reluctant or unconcerned about living a healthy lifestyle. Some people in this category may feel that, despite the increased health risks of a poor diet, the odds of poor health afflicting them specifically are low.[5] We live under the misconception that bad things always happen to someone else. After all, we all know someone who is obese or has had cancer or heart disease, but who would expect that someone to be you? This "that-could-never-happen-to-me" attitude is a common reason to avoid lifestyle changes, but, as you have learned so far, there are still many benefits to eating a healthy diet.

The more you think about the benefits of a healthy diet, the more you will be able to overcome the barriers that keep you from eating healthy foods. The key to making long-term change is being able to overcome the barriers and think more about the benefits. When the benefits start to overpower your excuses for not wanting to change, you will become more confident with your healthy eating behavior. As your confidence grows, you will eat better and enjoy more and more of the benefits.[2] In the following table, place a check mark by the benefits of good nutrition that you like; then check the reasons why you might struggle to eat good foods.⁶

Benefits of good nutrition	Reasons why it is hard to eat healthy foods
___ I feel better. ___ I can prevent many serious chronic diseases. ___ I can lose weight or maintain a healthy weight. ___ I feel like I'm doing the right thing.	___ I don't like the taste of healthy food. ___ Healthy food is expensive. ___ Unhealthy food is convenient, and I don't know how to cook.

Taste Trumps All

INSIDE THE ALDANA HOME ►►► *When I was a child, my mother used to cook brussels sprouts for dinner. I tried them, but they tasted terrible. I thought they were disgusting, but miraculously my mother (and others in the world) liked them. Twenty years later, I was just finishing graduate school and had completed a study about the great benefits of cruciferous vegetables (broccoli, cabbage, brussels sprouts, etc.). I figured that since I was now an adult with grown-up tastes, I should try to make brussels sprouts a part of my healthy diet. So I carefully selected some freshly picked ones, gently cooked and seasoned them, set the table, and prepared myself for a yummy meal. As I began chewing the first bite, the smell, taste, and texture circulated through my brain, and I was reminded once again that I still hated brussels sprouts. After 20 years, the taste hadn't changed, and I'm confident that I won't be giving them another chance. Taste alone will keep brussels sprouts from ever finding a place on my plate.*

Taste is one of the most important factors to consider when you try to adopt a healthy diet.¹ To most people, taste is more important than cost or ease of preparation. Children and young adults are especially influenced by the way foods taste, and our taste preferences often change over time. Foods that we preferred as children may not be as appealing to us now. You can even learn to like foods that you might not like right now.

For example, many people like the taste of whole milk. As we've learned, low-fat milk products should be part of your healthy diet, but, as most people know, there is a big difference in taste between whole-fat milk and low-fat or skim milk. To a whole-fat milk drinker, skim milk tastes like white water. To a skim-milk drinker, whole-fat milk tastes like cream or ice cream.

So how can a whole-fat milk drinker learn to drink healthier low-fat milk? You could try going cold turkey by swearing off whole-fat milk and never drinking it again, but for a less abrupt way, try drinking 2% milk. It has less than half the amount of fat as whole milk. After a few weeks of drinking 2%, try drinking 1%. In a month or two you will be ready for skim milk. It might take you a little time, but you can learn to like new foods. This is just one of several techniques you can use to learn to like the taste of healthier foods. And as you begin to eat healthier foods, your tastes will change.

Within all food groups, there are foods that you may or may not like. The trick is to find the ones you do like and make them a regular part of your diet. Alter the taste of your food by changing the way it is prepared. There are several good cookbooks that can help you quickly and easily prepare healthy meals. I suggest *5 a Day: The Better Health Cookbook* by Elizabeth Pivonka and *Quick & Healthy Recipes and Ideas: For People Who Say They Don't Have Time to Cook Healthy Meals* by Brenda J. Ponichtera. Kevin Vigilante and Mary Flynn have put together a great book about the Mediterranean diet called *Low-Fat Lies: High-Fat Frauds & the Healthiest Diet in the World*. These books contain time-tested recipes that are easy to use and healthy—and, best of all, they taste great.

There are also places online to get excellent free recipes. I recommend recipes from the National Institutes of Health (www.nhlbi.nih.gov/health/public/heart/other/ktb_recipebk/) and the American Heart Association (www.deliciousdecisions.org). With the knowledge you have gained from this book, you have the ability to evaluate any recipe and decide if it promotes good health. Try it and see if you like the taste. If you don't like the way it tastes, try something else. Experiment with different foods and different cooking techniques. Healthy foods like fruits, vegetables, whole grains, good fats, poultry, and milk taste great—experiment.

The research about healthy fats versus not-so-healthy fats is a radically different view of dietary fat and good health. If you are concerned with your weight, you want to keep an eye on the total amount of energy you consume. Dietary fat is high in calories, so you can't eat endless amounts of "healthy" dietary fat just because you've learned that they are full of heart healthy mono- and polyunsaturated fats. You can eat too much of a good thing. You can still enjoy some great tasting healthy fats and still control your weight.

There is a great big world of foods out there that are full of heart-healthy fats that taste great. The Mediterranean diet is high in healthy fats, and if you have ever eaten authentic Italian food, you know it tastes good. You can't use poor taste as an excuse not to eat foods that contain healthy fats. Here are more tips to help you enjoy healthy foods that taste good:

- Eat fruit with your breakfast every day. Nothing wakes up your mouth in the morning like a glass of fresh fruit juice or a piece of fresh fruit.
- Add more vegetables to your meals until vegetables gradually become the focus of the meal; try doubling the vegetable portion and reducing the red meat portion by half.
- Make substitutions—instead of adding lots of cheese to your baked potato, try adding green onions, chives, chili, or even a salad dressing made from healthy oils.
- There's nothing like a bowl of hot vegetable stew on a cold winter day. Add lots of vegetables and let it cook all day.
- Serve slices of fresh fruit as an appetizer to start a meal; fruit also makes a great dessert.
- Try different cooking techniques. Root vegetables, such as sweet potatoes, carrots, butternut squash, and acorn squash, can be oven roasted, cooked in the microwave, or steamed.
- Try stir-frying vegetables. It's pretty difficult to stir-fry vegetables and ruin them. Try cooking peppers, onions, pea pods, zucchini, and summer squash; add a little meat and rice, and you're ready for a great meal.
- Experiment with new cooking methods, spices, and ethnic foods. If you really want some great-tasting, healthy foods, try Thai food.

Cost

Does it cost more to eat healthy foods? Some would say yes and some no. If you live in Minneapolis in January and you want to eat fresh fruits and vegetables, the stores carry them, but they can be expensive out of season. Frozen, canned, or even dried vegetables are always available and are easy to prepare. In less than five minutes, you can open a bag of frozen vegetables and have them ready to eat. Best of all, you can purchase large quantities when they are on sale and keep them in your freezer. In many areas with more moderate climates, fresh fruits and vegetables are available year-round and are not expensive.

The cost of foods made from whole grains can be less than the cost of foods made with refined grains. Here is a list of whole-grain cereals. Wait for them to go on sale, and then buy enough for several months. Store them under your bed if you don't have room in your kitchen. Whole-grain breads can be frozen until you are ready to eat them.

General Mills	
Apple Cinnamon Cheerios Berry Burst Cheerios Honey Nut Cheerios Multi Grain Cheerios Oatmeal Crisp Cereals Total Wheaties Energy Crunch	Basic 4 Frosted Cheerios Milk 'n Cereal Bars Honey Nut Cheerios Nature Valley Low-Fat Fruit Granola Team Cheerios Total Brown Sugar & Oats Wheaties Raisin Bran
Quaker	
Life Cereal Honey Graham Life 100% Natural Granola, Oats & Honey Oatmeal Honey Nut Heaven	Cinnamon Life 100% Natural Granola, Oats, Honey & Raisins 100% Low-Fat Natural Granola Oatmeal Brown Sugar Bliss
Kellogg's	
Fruit Harvest Cereals Low-Fat Granola Mini-Wheats Cereals	Just Right Fruit & Nut Low-Fat Granola with Raisins Smart Start Cereals
Post	
Cinna-Cluster Raisin Bran Grape-Nuts Flakes Honey Nut Shredded Wheat Shredded Wheat Spoon Size Shredded Wheat	Frosted Shredded Wheat Great Grains Premium Raisin Bran Shredded Wheat 'n Bran
Breads, rolls	
Whole wheat bread Whole wheat English muffins Whole wheat rolls Tortilla chips, without trans fats	Whole wheat pitas Whole wheat bagels Whole wheat crackers Popcorn, without trans fats
Grains	
Whole wheat tortillas Whole wheat spaghetti Wild rice	Whole wheat macaroni Whole wheat noodles Bulgur

Table 12.1 Common whole-grain cereals and breads[7]

Fortunately, healthy foods are most often foods that are close to their natural form. A baked potato is much cheaper than french fries or potato chips. Beans, whole-grain cereals and breads, corn, potatoes, lentils, oatmeal, peas, apples, and other fruits and vegetables are full of fiber, phytochemicals, and energy, and these foods are almost always less expensive than their highly processed byproducts. Here are a few more tips to help keep costs down:

- Shop on a full stomach; you are likely to buy less food and make purchases based on good nutrition rather than the need to feed your hunger.
- Shop from a list and try to stick to it.
- There are a lot of coupons and discounts for highly processed foods, especially foods that are new or are being aggressively marketed. Use your discounts and coupons to pick healthy processed foods. Watch for advertisements in your local newspaper or in the mail from grocery stores offering sales on fresh fruits and vegetables. When they are on sale, buy as much as you and your family can eat and keep them handy.
- When you eat out, chances are you will receive an enormous plate filled with food. Next time you eat out, split a meal with a friend or partner. You get plenty of food for half the price, and you won't be pressured to clear your plate.
- When eating away from home, commit to eating healthy.
- Don't order an unhealthy dinner just because you are eating out. If someone else is paying, order the salmon!
- Start a small garden and plant only the foods you like to eat. You don't need lots of expensive gardening tools or fertilizer; work the soil, plant the vegetables, water them, and keep the weeds out.

Convenience

In 1995, 40% of the money Americans used to purchase food was spent on ready-to-eat foods away from home.[8] This includes fast food, food from restaurants, food from convenience stores, and any food purchased and eaten outside the home.[9] Foods eaten away from home are higher in energy and fat compared to foods eaten at home,[10] and foods purchased and eaten outside the home cost more. Despite the high calories and cost, foods eaten away from home are convenient. There are no dishes to clean or meals to prepare. The growth of convenience foods is probably due to the mobile nature of our society, the increasing amount of disposable income many people have, and the intense marketing efforts of food producers.

In 1998, Coca Cola spent $277 million on advertising.[11] One year later, McDonald's spent $571.7 million and Burger King spent $407.5 million to advertise their foods.[12,13] Contrast this amount of marketing with the $1 million spent by the National Cancer Institute to promote the 5-a-day fruit and vegetable message.[10] The entire nutrition education, evaluation, and demonstration budget of the U.S. Department of Agriculture was only 3% of what the food industry spent promoting fast foods that year.[10]

Most fruits are also foods of convenience, but they are not as highly promoted and cannot compete with the fast-food marketing efforts that permeate every aspect of our society. To help you make good nutrition choices, here is a list of ideas that can help you see that healthy foods can also be convenient foods:

- Use the microwave to prepare veggie-friendly meals, such as a baked potato with salsa and broccoli.
- Serve low-fat frozen yogurt with berries or peaches for a fast and easy dessert.
- Eat precut veggies with dip.
- Try apple or banana slices with peanut butter.
- Eat dried apricots and other dried fruits.
- Keep a bowl of washed fruit on your counter in plain sight where anyone can reach it.
- Try frozen or canned fruits and veggies.
- Try precut and washed fruits and vegetables if you prefer them fresh.
- Buy bagels when they are fresh and store them in the freezer. For lunch, grab a frozen wheat bagel when you leave the house in the morning and by the time you are ready to eat it, it will be thawed out.
- Take lunch rather than buying something.
- Go to www.fastfoodfacts.com, get a copy of the booklet *Nutrition in the Fast Lane,* and keep it in the glove box of your car. It contains the nutritional ingredients of foods sold in most fast food restaurants. Use it to pick foods low in trans and saturated fats.

Get Real—I've Got Kids!

It is hard enough for adults to adopt a healthy diet, but getting kids to eat healthy is an even greater challenge. Action for Healthy Kids is a nationwide initiative dedicated to improving the health of children through better nutrition and physical activity in schools. This group is composed of 50 state teams and a national coordinating and resource group, and it is helping children get good nutrition and exercise at school. At their Web site, www.actionforhealthykids.org, you will find great ideas for how to help your children eat healthy and be active. If you really want to make a difference, contact parents and concerned citizens in your state to see how you can encourage local school systems to provide a healthy food environment. Your community effort will improve the health of thousands of children and make your job as a parent even easier.

Probably the single most important thing you can do to get kids to live healthy lifestyles is to be a good example for them. In many ways, they grow up to be just like you. If they see you eating healthy foods and exercising, they learn to develop that same lifestyle. It may take a few years, but once they become adults, most will remember your example.

 INSIDE THE ALDANA HOME ▶▶▶ *Make funny faces on a plate by slicing apples, bananas, raisins, dried cranberries (Craisins), grapes, or any other fruit and then arranging them on a plate so they form a funny face or a picture. It doesn't take much effort, and I guarantee your kids will love it and ask you to do it again and again. In an ideal world, children would eat what they are supposed to. Sometimes you have to resort to subtle trickery and substitutions. My wife and I love to eat stir-fried vegetables. When we stir-fry, we sauté the meat first and set it aside. The adults eat stir-fried vegetables with rice and a little meat. The kids get the meat and a little rice, but instead of stir-fried vegetables, which they sometimes don't like, they get fresh carrots, snow peas, peas, and sometimes sliced pineapple. It's not worth fighting over.*

Kids also love to have fun with food, and as long as you make healthy foods fun, they will eat them. Here are a few time-tested ideas to try with your own children:

- Kids eat just about anything if it has peanut butter on it.
- Don't think of broccoli as a vegetable, think of it as a small tree. What child wouldn't like to eat a tree?
- Find alternatives to using food as a reward or bribe. Try stickers, hugs, or small toys, or simply say, "You did great!"
- For a bedtime snack, try whole wheat crackers, whole wheat toast, or a bowl of whole-grain cereal. Sliced fruit also makes a great snack.
- Kids warm up with hot chocolate made with skim milk and a piece of whole wheat toast.
- No kid can resist fresh strawberries or raspberries. (I grow raspberries in my garden, and I often see the kids picking and eating the berries on their own.)

- Make a parfait with fresh fruit, yogurt, and granola.
- Make waffles and pancakes with whole-grain flour.
- Improve any cereal by putting fruit on it.
- Make a vegetable soup bomb—hollow out a whole wheat roll, fill it with vegetable soup, and put the lid back on it.
- Insist that your children eat breakfast.
- Open a can of refried beans (low in saturated and trans fats), add a bit of cheese and maybe some fresh salsa, roll it in a whole wheat flour shell, and warm it up in the microwave. It's quick and tasty.
- Establish a general structure around meal and snack times and allow eating only at these times. Offer water, fruits and vegetables, or other healthy snacks if kids are still hungry between eating times.
- Eat meals as a family as often as possible.
- Limit soda, punch, and flavored waters to special occasions.
- Teach your kids to cook healthy meals.
- Set limits on TV and computer game time. After one to two hours, it is time to play something else, preferably something that involves physical activity.

For more ideas on how to get your children to like healthy foods, I recommend these two books: *Quick Meals for Healthy Kids and Busy Parents: Wholesome Family Recipes in 30 Minutes or Less from Three Leading Child Nutrition Experts* by Sandra K. Nissenberg, Margaret L. Bogle, and Audrey C. Wright and *Healthy Treats and Super Snacks for Kids* by Jeff MacNelly. Be patient with your children; if you are making lifestyle changes for yourself, don't expect them to do the same. As you start to make changes, they will see the benefits you are experiencing, and they will slowly decide to join you.

Expect Setbacks

Pretend it is the middle of January. At the beginning of the year you made some New Year's resolutions, and you've been doing great for two weeks. Perhaps the demands from work or school have changed, you have a new boyfriend or girlfriend, you got the flu, or for some other reason, your social situation changed. You may be emotionally upset or just stressed out. One night you decide to eat six doughnuts and a big box of french fries. After all, you deserve it. This momentary setback to your healthy diet is a relapse to your previous eating habits. Everyone has setbacks—this is a common part of the behavior change process.[14] Since it happens to everyone, the best thing to do is to prepare for the time when it happens, realize what is happening, and then get back to your healthy diet.

Use these momentary weaknesses to strengthen your resolve; don't allow them to create feelings of guilt and negative emotions. Even the most devoted person occasionally slips. The sight of food, social situations, hunger, and taste perception may tempt you to abandon your efforts. If you don't know how to cope, you start eating poor foods, your confidence decreases, and you eventually lose your motivation and control of eating. If, on the other hand, you have some tools to help you cope with high-risk situations, you can prevent mistakes. Success increases your self-confidence and helps you have long-term control of your food choices.[15]

> ## Rome wasn't built in a single day, and your lifetime of eating habits can't be altered overnight.

Don't allow yourself to get into situations where you are tempted. You might need to change your environment. If your home is free of problem foods, you won't be tempted. Avoid situations where you know unhealthy foods will be served. Don't wait until you are starving to find some place to eat—you will settle for unhealthy foods just to satisfy your hunger.

Think about your food triggers—situations or settings that precede your weak moments. Try to recognize your triggers and avoid them if possible. Common triggers include the enticement to eat food while watching TV, the habit of eating just before bed, the tendency to eat because you are stressed, the routine of walking by a doughnut shop every day, or the tendency to stuff yourself every time you eat out just to make sure you get your money's worth. Structure your day to include opportunities to eat healthy foods. Take your lunch instead of eating from vending machines.

You have a better chance of avoiding relapse if you have social support. If you haven't already, share this book with your family, peers, work colleagues, and friends. Give them their own copies so they are better educated and more willing to help you and themselves aggressively stick to a healthy lifestyle.[16] Few things help you more than good friends or loved ones who want you to succeed.

Get Out of Your Comfort Zone

It is time to get serious about changing your nutrition. That means you need to set a goal and commit to doing it.[17] Set a goal that is relatively simple and easy to accomplish, or stretch yourself and get a little more aggressive. The Steps to a Healthier U.S. Initiative (www.healthierus.gov) has put together a great list of very simple steps you can take to improve your nutrition. Read the list below and see if there are some steps you can use as simple goals for yourself. You have to start sometime, so pick one of these or make up one of your own.

Simple Nutrition Goals

Use fat-free milk instead of whole milk.
Drink water before a meal.
Eat leaner red meat and poultry.
Eat only half of your dessert.
Avoid food portions larger than your fist.
Increase the fiber in your diet.
Drink diet soda, or try to drink more water.
Eat off of smaller plates.
Don't eat late at night.
Skip seconds.
Skip buffets.
Grill, steam, or bake instead of frying.
Use vegetable oils instead of solid fats.
More carrots, less cake.
Don't skip meals.
Eat more celery sticks.
Keep to a regular eating schedule.
Choose fruit for dessert.
Consume alcoholic beverages in moderation, if at all.
Share a restaurant meal with a friend.
Grill vegetables.
Eat before grocery shopping.
Choose a checkout line without a candy display.
Make a grocery list before you shop.
Buy 100% fruit juices instead of soda and sugary drinks.
Flavor foods with herbs, spices, and other low-fat seasonings.
Remove skin from poultry before cooking to lower fat content.
Eat before you get too hungry.
Don't skip breakfast.
Stop eating when you are full.
Snack on fruits and vegetables.

Top your favorite cereal with apples or bananas.
Try brown rice or whole-wheat pasta.
Include several servings of whole-grain food daily.
When eating out, choose a small- or medium-sized portion.
If main dishes are too big, choose an appetizer or a side dish instead.
Ask for salad dressing "on the side."
Try a green salad instead of fries.
Eat sweet foods in small amounts.
Drink lots of water.
Limit yourself to one "treat" a day.

If you think you are ready to be more aggressive about improving your diet, here is a list of achievable nutrition goals that you might want to try:

- I will eat at least five servings of fruits and/or vegetables every day for a week.
- Half of the grains I eat during a seven-day period will be whole grains.
- Instead of red meat, I will eat fish, poultry, or eggs.
- I will read the labels on every food I eat for a week to determine if they contain trans fats.
- I will include fruit and whole grains in my breakfast every day for a week.
- Make your own goal.

After you have decided on a goal, write it down using the contract form below. After all, a goal not written is only a wish.

My Goal:

_____

_____

_____

To demonstrate how committed you are, share this goal with someone and sign it.

Signature:_____Date:_____

The last thing you have to do is to track your progress. If your goal requires daily effort, keep track of your progress by marking off each day on a calendar. If you relapse, don't beat yourself up over it. Just forget about it and get back to keeping your goal. If you have been successful for a while, it may be time to start on another goal. For more motivation, go back and reread the information about how your efforts will transform your life.

Nutritious meal and snack ideas

It is easy to get good nutrition if you eat three meals a day and have only a couple of snacks. Try some of these ideas:

For breakfast try . . .
a fruit smoothie or glass of juice
an omelet with fresh peppers, onions, and tomatoes
a whole wheat pancake or waffle topped with fruit
a toasted whole wheat bagel topped with low-fat cream cheese and tomato or bell
   peppers
some whole-grain cereal topped with fruit

Lunch is easy with . . .
a salad
a sandwich with whole wheat bread, sliced turkey, and lots of fresh veggies
some vegetable soup with chips that have no trans fats
a veggie pizza

Dinner can end the day with . . .
vegetable lasagna
stir-fried vegetables with meat and rice
pasta tossed with vegetables
salad topped with grilled salmon or chicken
barbecued chicken with fresh vegetables and fruit
trans fat-free tortilla chips, fresh salsa, and guacamole

Take It Slow and Easy

You've been eating the same way for years; you shouldn't expect to change your diet in a flash. Rome wasn't built in a single day, and your lifetime of eating habits can't be altered overnight. The process of adopting good nutrition behaviors takes a long time, sometimes years, so be patient. Pick one thing to work on for a while; when you have it mastered, move on to something else.

Celebrate your successes by rewarding yourself with non-food-related treats. If you have a favorite hobby or activity, consider using this as a reward for doing well. Use rewards that link some of your favorite things with eating healthy foods. Eating is a pleasurable part of life. Rather than thinking about breaking bad habits, think about establishing good ones. Don't concentrate just on eliminating processed foods from your diet; first add three more servings of fresh fruits and vegetables to your diet. You'll likely find that the unhealthy foods in your diet slowly start disappearing.

POINTS TO REMEMBER

- Keep thinking about the benefits of eating a healthy diet.

- Healthy foods can be tasty too. Try different recipes, make small changes, and don't be afraid to experiment.

- There is little difference in the cost of eating healthy foods versus unhealthy ones.

- Convenience is not really a barrier to good nutrition. There are lots of healthy foods that are "fast."

- Kids can learn to like healthy foods. You need to set a good example and be creative.

- Everyone experiences failures and setbacks. Be patient and take small steps.

CALORIES ►

PORTION SIZE ►

SNACK FOODS ►

SODA ►

GENES ►

SKILLS ►

MOTIVATION ►

GOOD CHOICES ►

COMMITMENT ►

EXERCISE ►

WEIGH OFTEN ►

HEALTHY EMOTIONAL STATE ►

CHAPTER

/13

Weight Loss:
A Healthy Lifestyle Side Effect

I've been on a constant diet for the last two decades.
I've lost a total of 789 pounds. By all accounts,
I should be hanging from a charm bracelet.
—Erma Bombeck (1927–1996)

NEXT TIME YOU ARE IN A CROWD, LOOK AROUND. Six out of every 10 adults in the United States today are overweight or obese.[1] Three out of every 10 men and 4 out of every 10 women are trying to lose weight, and 3 out of every 10 adults are actively trying to maintain weight.[2,3] Americans know they are overweight and are tying to do something about it. This preoccupation with weight is also occurring among people in Australia, England, Portugal, India, and every other Westernized nation in the world. Excessive body weight is a lifestyle problem that knows no borders.

In the past 10 years, researchers have studied healthy lifestyles to see if they can be effective in treating common health problems such as high blood cholesterol, blood pressure, diabetes, and other conditions. Individuals with symptoms or risks of chronic diseases were recruited to participate in these lifestyle studies. Many study participants were asked to take part in a lifestyle change program (similar to what I have outlined in this book) instead of taking medication. Different variations of life-style programs were tried. You may have heard of the Diabetes Prevention Program, the Dean Ornish Heart Disease Reversing Program, the

Coronary Health Improvement Program, or even the Dietary Approaches to Stop Hypertension (DASH) diet. Other lifestyle change interventions didn't have specific names, but they all included regular exercise and some variation of a prudent diet. None of them was designed as a weight-control program; they were all hoping to correct a specific health condition. Interestingly, every single study had one common result: subjects who were in the lifestyle modification groups lost weight.

Besides improvements in blood pressure, subjects in the PREMIER blood pressure study lost 13 pounds on average.[4] Obese men who participated in a study in Italy not only experienced significant improvements in erectile dysfunction, but also lost an average of 33 pounds after two years.[5] Study participants in the Diabetes Prevention Program dramatically reduced their chances of becoming diabetic, and in addition, they lost 7% of their body weight (or about 12 pounds on average) and kept the weight off for several years.[6] Whichever study you consider, if it had lifestyle intervention as a treatment, weight loss was an outcome; weight loss was not the primary focus of any of these studies, but it happened anyway because weight loss is a side effect of a healthy lifestyle.

This makes sense because a healthy lifestyle includes regular physical activity and a prudent diet (which has fewer calories than what most people normally eat). Obviously there are considerable variations in how these studies were conducted, but the common theme among them all is that weight loss and healthy weight maintenance are possible with lifestyle modification. It may be easier to eat a prudent diet and accept it as a way of living than it is to stay with a Western-type diet that requires you to carefully select which foods to reduce or eliminate in order to cut calories. With a healthy lifestyle you can eat until you are satisfied while still preventing chronic diseases and maintaining a healthy weight.[7]

Our Culture of Consumption

Excessive body weight is a problem for most Americans for two main reasons: (1) we have a culture that encourages excessive food consumption, and (2) we live in a society that discourages physical activity.[8] Kelly Brownell, a psychologist at the Yale Center for Eating and Weight Disorders who specializes in weight control, has labeled our unhealthy culture "a toxic environment."[9] Those are pretty strong words, but as you will see, they may be appropriate. Chapters 9–11 were devoted to addressing the part of this toxic environment that discourages physical activity. Let's see how this same environment affects the way we view food and eating.

If you recall, both men and women eat more calories per day now than at any other time since researchers began collecting data on this subject. As the average caloric intake has increased, the percent of calories that come from fat has decreased from 45% to 32% (see chapter 7). These two changes in food consumption appear to be in opposition to each other—on the one hand, we are eating more calories, but on the other hand, the percent of our food that comes from fat has decreased.

In reality, there is no opposition here. While the overall percentage of calories from fat has decreased, the total amount of fat, as measured in grams per day, has increased. We now eat more total calories than ever before, and even though fewer of these calories come from fat on a percentage basis, the total amount of fat we eat every day has increased.[10,11] Between 1970 and 1996, the amount of fats and oils added to the U.S. food supply increased by 22%.[12] During this same time period, cheese consumption increased from 11 pounds per person per year to 28 pounds per person per year, an increase of 146%.[12] Most of the extra cheese comes from tacos, nachos, pizza, and other fast foods, and the extra fat in our diets is mostly saturated and trans fats.[12]

One of the most obvious changes to occur in our culture is the amount of food served when we eat out. Of all the meals Americans eat, 27% are eaten outside the home,[12] and at least part of the blame for America's weight problem can be placed on the expanding portions offered at restaurants. Since the late 1970s, there has been a gradual and steady increase in the number of large-sized food portions served at restaurants. It used to be that you could eat at a restaurant and get your food served on a plate; now it comes on a platter.[13] Figure 13.1 shows the increase in the number of larger-sized food portions introduced by fast food establishments and restaurants since the 1970s.

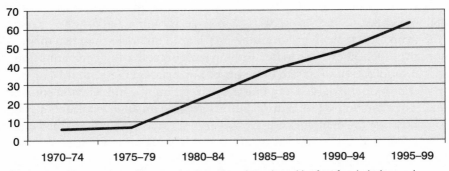

Figure 13.1 The number of larger-sized portions introduced by fast food chains and restaurants[13]

These large-sized servings can make you feel like royalty with names like "King size" and "Queen size." At 7-Eleven you can purchase a 16-ounce Gulp soda drink. Not to be outdone, there is also the 32-ounce Big Gulp and the 64-ounce Double Gulp with a whopping 800 calories. In the 1950s, McDonald's only had one size of french fries; a 1950s-size order of fries is today's small. If you don't want the small, you can get a medium, large, or super size. You can even super size your whole meal. Why settle for a McDonald's Big Mac when you can have a Big Xtra with cheese or even a Monster Mac made with four, instead of two, 1.6-ounce beef patties?

Candy bars, chips, cookies, and other snack foods are also sold in extra large sizes. The larger size usually means you get more food for your money. Despite the economic savings, the larger sizes also tend to encourage us to eat more.[14,15] Unless eating more is countered with increased physical activity, the result is weight gain.

The marketing pressure from food producers is intense and often misleading. Kids who visit the official Web site of Butterfinger candy bars (www.butterfinger.com) can learn how Butterfinger candy bars are good for you. Here is the exact text from their Web site:

- Crunching into a Butterfinger is a good workout. (For your jaw.)
- Lifting the Butterfinger to your mouth numerous times is a good workout. (For your jaw.)
- Carrying a lot of Butterfingers around is a good full body workout. (Providing that you're carrying around a big crate. And always lift with the knees.)

The Soda Factor

Another source of increased calories is soda. The typical American drank 34.7 gallons of soda in 1987. Ten years later the amount had increased to 44.4 gallons per person per year. This is an average, meaning that for every person who drinks less than 44 gallons, someone is drinking more than that—teenage boys especially appear to be drinking more soda than average.[16]

In moderation, soda can be a part of any prudent diet, but the key is moderation; the Double Gulp might be stretching the moderation envelope just a bit. Soft-drink manufacturers are also pushing extremely hard to make soda the drink of choice for everyone, especially school-aged children. Their aggressive marketing and advertising tactics to school-aged children through school districts influences children to drink soda, which is not helping America's weight problem.

Blaming Genes for Your Tight Jeans

The shape of your body, where you store fat in your body, your height, and, to a small degree, your weight may be predetermined by the genes you inherit from your parents. If your parents store fat in and around the chest and abdomen, you will most likely store your fat in the same places. If you are female and your mother carries her body fat on her waist and hips, you are likely to do the same. Fat deposition location is very much determined by genetics. However, the amount of fat you carry is more a result of your environment and lifestyle than genetics. There are some genes that can cause excessive weight gain, but these are very rare.

The increase in obesity in the United States has occurred in just two or three decades, with very little change in the genetic makeup of the U.S. population. Such a dramatic increase cannot be due to genetics because the genetic pool of the entire population cannot change in 20 years. Only a change in food and physical activity behaviors can cause such a relatively rapid change in weight. It appears that our toxic food environment, not genetics, should bear much of the blame.

On a Diet, Off a Diet

When it all boils down, weight loss is nothing more than balancing energy from food with energy expended by the body.

weight change = calories in − calories out

This equation is the energy balance theory of weight control. When the number of calories you eat is greater than the number of calories you expend, the extra calories are stored as body fat and your weight increases. During the holidays, when food is plentiful and physical activity is often replaced with more sedentary activities, the amount of calories people expend does not keep up with their food intake and they gain weight. No wonder New Year's resolutions are often centered on weight loss.

With so many people struggling to lose weight in our "I want it now" American culture, it is not surprising that there are so many different weight-loss methods available. Newspapers, magazines, television, and e-mail spam all promote fast, effective weight-loss programs. And these programs must be selling well—the weight-loss industry is a 33-billion-dollar-a-year industry.

Among Americans who are actively trying to lose weight, the methods they use most often are as follows[2]:

60% eat fewer calories
51% eat less fat
53% exercise more
10% skip meals
5% eat food supplements
3% join weight-loss programs
2% take weight-loss pills
a few fast for 24-hour periods

Surprisingly, only one-fourth of those who are trying to lose weight combine eating fewer calories with exercise, a combination that dramatically increases the odds of long-term weight loss.[2,3]

With so many people trying to lose weight and so many people trying to maintain a healthy weight, one has to wonder if any of these methods actually work. The best weight-loss programs are designed to help individuals reduce caloric intake and increase physical activity. They do this by providing the skills and motivation necessary to make good nutrition choices and to stay physically active. But do they work? Can people successfully lose weight and keep it off over the long term?

Weight loss followed by weight gain is the most common result for most people who participate in weight-loss programs. Despite what you may have seen or experienced, most individuals who lose weight experience the same process: weight is lost when diet and exercise efforts are most consistent, followed by a slow and gradual regaining of most of the lost weight. Figure 13.2 shows what happens to the typical weight-loss program participant.

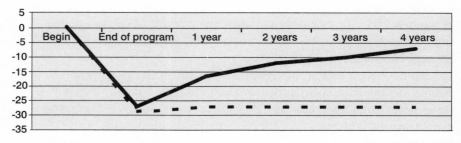

Figure 13.2 The solid line shows the typical results of weight-loss program participants in pounds. The dotted line would be ideal—lose weight and keep it off for years.[17]

As long as an individual adheres to caloric restriction and regular exercise, weight loss occurs, regardless of whether individuals are able to do this on their own or if they are participating in a structured weight-loss program. Weight loss is directly related to the intensity of the weight-loss efforts and the length of time the efforts are made. So why do people regain the weight? Some have proposed that the body has a predetermined weight that it naturally tries to maintain.[18] This means that after weight loss, the body might try to gain weight until it reaches some predetermined weight or fixed set point. However, there is a more probable explanation for why so many people regain lost weight.

When people use the word *diet* in relation to weight loss, it usually means a change in the normal foods people eat. We "go on a diet" when we start the eating behavior that we hope will help us lose weight—this usually means fewer calories. Not surprisingly, weight is lost. But after the weight has been lost, the diet that caused the weight loss slowly begins to revert to its previous form as we slowly go "off" the diet.[19]

The regaining of body weight, illustrated in Figure 13.2, is caused by failure to permanently change the behaviors that caused the excess weight in the first place. With time, many dieters slowly begin to exercise less or eat more calories until their diet and physical activity habits are similar to the ones they had when they first gained the weight. It would appear that successful long-term weight loss is directly linked to food and exercise behavior. To clarify this point, it is necessary to check in with the real winners in the weight-loss battle, the ones who have lost weight and kept it off for at least five years.

The Weight-Control Masters

The National Weight Loss Registry contains information on thousands of women and men who have lost weight and kept it off, individuals who used to be obese and are now at a healthy weight. Of the people listed in the registry, 800 have lost an average of 66 pounds and have been successful in keeping at least half of that weight off for five years. I like to call these people the "weight-control masters." Individuals enrolled in the registry periodically complete questionnaires about their success at losing weight, current weight-maintenance strategies, and other health-related behaviors. This information is later analyzed to see if there are common characteristics among participants.[20-25]

Nine out of 10 of the weight-control masters used calorie restriction and regular physical activity as their method for both losing weight and maintaining weight loss. Almost all of them controlled their food calories by limiting intake of certain types or classes of foods. Others limited quantities of food in general and counted calories. Almost all reported that they exercised at home, and about one-third said they exercised with a group or a friend.

One of the most telling pieces of information that comes from these weight-control masters is the fact that three-quarters of them reported that there was a triggering event or incident that preceded their successful efforts to lose weight. These events included medical triggers (e.g., varicose veins, sleep disturbances, low back pain, fatigue and tiredness, aching legs, diabetes). Other triggers were more emotional in nature—"My husband was worried about my weight and health" or "My 25th anniversary was approaching, and I wanted to look good for it." Whether the trigger was physical or emotional, it served as a strong motivational call to action.

Weight-control masters also ate at fast food restaurants less than once a week, and at non-fast food restaurants 2.5 times per week on average. This suggests that they ate the majority of their meals at home, and meals eaten at home generally have fewer calories and are lower in fat.

For most, weight loss was preceded by some trigger—a strong motivational call to action.

Physical activity was also very important for both weight loss and maintenance and appears to be a major part of their success. The amount of energy the masters expended in physical activity each week would be equal to walking four miles every day. That is slightly more than the overall recommendation for Americans to get 30 minutes or more of moderate-intensity activity every day. All of these masters had to gradually increase their activity until they could comfortably maintain their daily exercise efforts.

The masters must be normal people like you and me, because 9 out of 10 had tried to lose weight before and failed. When asked to compare their successful weight-loss experience with previous weight-loss failures, most said they had greater social reasons, health reasons, or both. Whatever their past experience had been, this time they were more committed to making permanent lifestyle changes.

What I like most about the masters is the benefits they report. A majority of them said that because of their weight loss, they had improved quality of life, increased energy, greater mobility, better general mood, increased self-confidence, more interactions with members of the opposite sex, better job performance, more participation in hobbies, and more interactions with family members. It would appear that besides the obvious improvements in physical appearance and health, successful weight loss can provide dramatic improvements in quality of life.[20]

So what should you take away from the experience of the weight-control masters? First, the weight-control masters all volunteered to join the registry; there may be many individuals not in the registry who use many of the same weight-loss strategies and fail to maintain their weight loss. Second, even though the weight-control masters give us some great examples, we still don't know the best way to maintain long-term weight loss. That said, the weight-control masters give us some great tips on how to have long-term success:

- Eat fewer calories. This can be accomplished by reducing the amount of food you eat and eating foods that are more likely to promote good health. Most of the masters switched to low-fat foods and ate less sugar and sweets and more fruits and vegetables.
- Exercise every day. Most exercised for an hour a day. If you really want to keep the weight off, you will have to make exercise part of your everyday life.
- Weigh yourself every week. Set a weight limit and don't exceed that limit.
- Cultivate social support. Friends, family, and even pets can provide emotional support and encouragement to start and stick with an active, healthy lifestyle.
- Commit to doing it. Make a decision to change your lifestyle. If you have a good reason to change (a trigger), use it to focus your efforts and solidify your determination.
- Find your approach. Everybody has a slightly different approach. Even though there were some common characteristics among many of the weight-control masters, others did it their own way. One size does not fit all when it comes to successful weight loss.

In 2002, *Consumer Reports*[26] invited readers to complete a survey about their weight-loss efforts. Of the 32,000 individuals who responded, 25% said they had been able to lose at least 10% of their body weight and keep it off for one year. The weight-loss method of choice for this group was, once again, eating less and exercising more. Most of them did not use commercial weight-loss programs and instead of lowering the amount of fat they were eating, many lowered the number of carbohydrates in their diet. The low-carbohydrate diet is a popular approach to weight loss that deserves a little more discussion.

Diet, Diet, Who's Got the Diet?

Despite all the research conducted on weight-loss programs, we still do not know what the best diet strategy is.[27] The most popular diet at the time this book was written was the Atkins diet. Before the Atkins diet became popular, there was the South Beach diet, the Zone diet, the Scarsdale diet, the Cabbage Soup diet, the Hollywood 48-Hour Miracle diet, the Grapefruit diet, the Negative Calorie diet, the 3-Day Diet, and many, many more. Regardless of the name and the guidelines of each of these diets, they all have two things in common—a lot of hype and calorie restriction. These diets have lower calories because when you follow them, you will be cutting something out of your normal diet. And that something is likely to be fat, carbohydrates, alcohol, or protein.

Based on what we have discussed in the nutrition chapters of this book, you have enough understanding of nutrition and health to be able to determine if a diet is going to promote good health or possibly lead to poor health. For example, let's take a closer look at the Atkins diet, a low-carbohydrate diet.

The Atkins diet promotes a low-carbohydrate diet. Dieters on the program are encouraged to eat no more than 20 grams of carbohydrates per day—one slice of bread has 20 grams. They can eat unlimited amounts of animal foods (meat, fowl, fish, and shellfish); unlimited eggs; 4 ounces of cheese; 2 cups of salad vegetables; and 1 cup of other vegetables per day. After a few months they are allowed to gradually reintroduce some carbohydrates into their diet. Since this diet became popular, nutritionists have lamented it because they know it goes contrary to much of the science that shows the possibly harmful effects of red meat and saturated and trans fats. It was believed that a diet high in saturated and trans fats would increase blood cholesterol (and thus increase heart disease risk) and all that red meat would increase cancer risk.

At the present time, research on the Atkins diet fails to paint such a gloomy picture. After one year, blood cholesterol for dieters on the Atkins diet did not worsen; on the contrary, it improved by a small margin.[28,29] Several studies compared the effects of the Atkins diet with a standard low-fat diet.[30-34] In general, people on both diets lost weight initially, with the low-carbohydrate participants losing slightly more weight than the other dieters did. After one year there was essentially no difference in weight loss between the two groups.

The graph in Figure 13.2 charts the results of a low-fat diet, but if the same study were done with a low-carbohydrate diet, the graph would look pretty much the same. Everything goes well during the initial weight-loss period, but weight is regained over time because the diet is not maintained

---

Everything goes well during the initial weight-loss period, but weight is regained over time because the diet is not maintained nor has physical activity been incorporated into everyday life. The biggest predictor of long-term weight-loss success is the adoption of a healthy lifestyle.

---

nor has physical activity been incorporated into everyday life. It doesn't matter if you choose a low-fat or low-carbohydrate diet; after about a year the results of both diets are about the same.[29] Some would argue that there are differences in how the different diets can delay hunger, but these variations are very subjective and not large. The biggest predictor of long-term weight-loss success is the adoption of a healthy lifestyle.

In his last book,[35] Dr. Atkins refined his diet to include a more health-oriented approach. In it he encourages less red meat and more tofu, nuts, and legumes; healthy oils; and more low-carbohydrate vegetables and fruits. These changes do much to improve the health-promoting effects of the diet.

As long as Americans are intent on finding a quick fix to long-term lifestyle problems, there will continue to be a neverending supply of fad diets vying for their moment in the limelight. Hopefully there will also be an ever-increasing group of people who realize that the only long-term solution is a healthy lifestyle.

How Much Should You Weigh?

In chapter 4 you used the body mass index chart to determine your body mass index (BMI). Here is the same chart:

Body Mass Index Chart

Weight (lbs)

Height	120	130	140	150	160	170	180	190	200	210	220	230	240	250	260	270	280	>290
4'5"	30	33	35	38	40	43	45	48	50	53	55	58	60	63	65	68	70	73
4'6"	29	31	34	36	39	41	43	46	48	51	53	55	58	60	63	65	68	70
4'7"	28	30	33	35	37	40	42	44	46	49	51	53	56	58	60	63	65	67
4'8"	27	29	31	34	36	38	40	43	45	47	49	52	54	56	58	61	63	65
4'9"	26	28	30	32	35	37	39	41	43	45	48	50	52	54	56	58	61	63
4'10"	25	27	29	31	33	36	38	40	42	44	46	48	50	52	54	56	59	61
4'11"	24	26	28	30	32	34	36	38	40	42	44	46	48	50	53	55	57	59
5'0"	23	25	27	29	31	33	35	37	39	41	43	45	47	49	51	53	55	57
5'1"	23	25	26	28	30	32	34	36	38	40	42	43	45	47	49	51	53	55
5'2"	22	24	26	27	29	31	33	35	37	38	40	42	44	46	48	49	51	53
5'3"	21	23	25	27	28	30	32	34	35	37	39	41	43	44	46	48	50	51
5'4"	21	22	24	26	27	29	31	33	34	36	38	39	41	43	45	46	48	50
5'5"	20	22	23	25	27	28	30	32	33	35	37	38	40	42	43	45	47	48
5'6"	19	21	23	24	26	27	29	31	32	34	36	37	39	40	42	44	45	47
5'7"	19	20	22	23	25	27	28	30	31	33	34	36	38	39	41	42	44	45
5'8"	18	20	21	23	24	26	27	29	30	32	33	35	36	38	40	41	43	44
5'9"	18	19	21	22	24	25	27	28	30	31	32	34	35	37	38	40	41	43
5'10"	17	19	20	22	23	24	26	27	29	30	32	33	34	36	37	39	40	42
5'11"	17	18	20	21	22	24	25	26	28	29	31	32	33	35	36	38	39	40
6'0"	16	18	19	20	22	23	24	26	27	28	30	31	33	34	35	37	38	39
6'1"	16	17	18	20	21	22	24	25	26	28	29	30	32	33	34	36	37	38
6'2"	15	17	18	19	21	22	23	24	26	27	28	30	31	32	33	35	36	37
6'3"	15	16	17	19	20	21	22	24	25	26	27	29	30	31	32	34	35	36
6'4"	15	16	17	18	19	21	22	23	24	26	27	28	29	30	32	33	34	35
6'5"	14	15	17	18	19	20	21	23	24	25	26	27	28	30	31	32	33	34
6'6"	14	15	16	17	18	20	21	22	23	24	25	27	28	29	30	31	32	34
6'7"	14	15	16	17	18	19	20	21	23	24	25	26	27	28	29	30	32	33
6'8"	13	14	16	16	18	19	20	21	22	23	24	25	26	27	29	30	31	32
6'9"	13	14	15	16	17	18	19	20	21	23	24	25	26	27	28	29	30	31
6'10"	13	14	15	16	17	18	19	20	21	22	23	24	25	26	27	28	29	30

| Underweight | Ideal weight (low risk) | Overweight (moderate risk) | Obese (high risk) |

Ideal weight is associated with a BMI of less than 25. You can use this information to determine a healthy weight that you can use as a goal. Since your height isn't going to change, find your height in the chart and follow the row over until you reach a BMI of 24; then move up the chart until you find the weight that corresponds with the BMI of 24. For example, for a woman who is 5'8" tall, the weight associated with a BMI of 24 is 160 pounds. This is the weight that is at the upper end of the ideal weight range. There is nothing magical about having a BMI of 24 versus a BMI of 25, although health risks do decrease with lower weight. This method of determining a healthy weight works for most people, but not all. If you have a large frame, you are always going to weigh more than the ideal weight shown in the chart. This is also true if you are very muscular.

If you are obese or overweight, another way to identify a good weight-loss goal is to plan on losing 5–10% of your body weight. Just multiply your current weight by 0.05 or 0.1 to see how many pounds you should lose. This amount of weight is small enough to be achievable and is also associated with improvements in diabetes, blood pressure, and blood cholesterol. If you are successful losing this much weight, you can always lose another 5%. Ideal weight is an individual decision and must be realistic. When you are deciding what weight to strive for, consider your lifestyle, health status, cultural and social values, and personal desires.

Why Exercise Makes a Big Difference

There are a few specifics about exercise that may help you stay committed once you learn about them. Weight can be lost with dieting alone. Figure 13.3 shows the results of some dieters who did nothing more than reduce the number of calories they were eating. They lost about 20 pounds—half the weight was from fat and the other half was lean tissue or muscle. Another group used only exercise to reduce their weight. They lost about 15 pounds total and actually gained a couple of pounds of muscle. A third group did both. This group lost more total weight than the others,

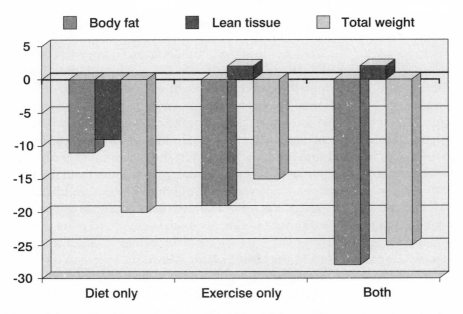

Figure 13.3 The effect of diet only, exercise only, and both on fat, muscle, and total body weight[36,37]

lost considerably more total body fat, and gained 2 pounds of muscle—they saved their muscle and even added a little to it.

This data provides significant information about the importance of combining exercise and calorie restriction. Muscle requires energy just to exist—each pound of muscle expends 30–60 calories per day, even if you don't use it for exercise. When you are sleeping, your muscles continue to use energy, and this helps burn calories. Muscle also gives you the necessary strength to be more physically active and to do activities that improve your quality of life.

The exercise recommendations for good health and the recommendations for starting a weight-loss program are the same—every adult should accumulate 30 minutes or more of moderate-intensity physical activity on most, preferably all, days of the week, and even more activity is better. For weight loss, a gradual increase in the amount of exercise is recommended. If you are overweight and sedentary and thinking about becoming physically active, it is always a good idea to get clearance from your physician.[27] Ideally, individuals who are trying to lose and maintain a healthy weight should do more than 30 minutes of activity every day; 60 minutes is better. That's how much the weight-control masters did. Besides improved body weight, this level of activity gives you a host of other benefits.

Slow and Steady Wins the Race

Extra weight can take years to appear. You don't get fat in just a few short weeks, so you shouldn't try to lose it all in that amount of time. The faster you lose the weight, the quicker the weight will come back. Rapid weight loss can be followed by larger and sometimes more rapid weight gain. In a very large national study, participants were at or above their original weight after two years when they used very low-calorie diets to lose weight.[38] When compared to those who lost the weight more gradually, there was no difference after three years. Reduce total calories from food by 500–1,000 calories a day to lose one to two pounds per week. In addition to reducing total energy intake, it is recommended that you reduce dietary fat intake to less than 30% of your total energy intake.[27]

Healthy Emotional State before Healthy Body Weight

For some, depression or family problems can make the desire and motivation to work toward a healthy weight difficult. For those who struggle with these issues, counseling and psychotherapy can help them think through their concerns and provide new perspectives and solutions to difficult problems. Sometimes medication is needed as part of treatment. Once these is-sues have been resolved, individuals are more likely to understand what food means to them and work through the problems that lead to overeating.[39]

Weigh Yourself Often

Use a bathroom scale at least once a week to measure your body weight. The scale won't lie. Use it to see how you are doing. If your weight goes up one month, don't be concerned unless it continues to increase. Set a reason-able maximum body weight and don't allow yourself to go above that weight.

Don't Buy Bigger Clothes

When weight gain causes your clothes to feel tighter, the wrong thing to do is buy bigger clothes. You can get comfortable clothes again by losing the extra weight. Tight-fitting clothes can act as a reminder of your need to lose those extra pounds.

Know Your Hunger Triggers

Studies of eating behavior show that we eat according to the different hunger triggers we encounter every day. Triggers are stimuli that make us want to eat. Time of day, the smell of food, stress, boredom, grocery shopping, and even advertisements can be triggers. Successful weight maintenance requires conscious identification and control of hunger triggers. By identifying your hunger triggers, you can learn to eat when you are hungry and not just because it's noon.

Eat on the Defensive

Here are some ideas to help you defend against eating too much.

- Do nothing else while eating; just enjoy your food. If you habitually watch TV while you eat, you might be tempted to eat each time you turn on the TV.
- Stop eating when you are full. When you eat out, you don't have to try to get your money's worth just because you are eating out. Take some home in a doggy bag.
- Don't eat everything on your plate (even though your mother told you to). The last thing most of us need is to load a plate with food and eat everything on it.
- When eating out, chose smaller portions or share your meal with someone. A couple of appetizers are just about as much food as an entrée.

- Don't bring problem foods home. Out of sight, out of mind.
- You don't have to have dessert at every meal. If you do need a dessert, have a small serving or some fruit.
- When you are done eating dinner, remove the serving dishes from the table so you aren't tempted to keep eating.

You Already Have Weight-Loss Goals

Whether you are trying to improve your health, prevent chronic disease, or lose weight, the physical activity and nutrition goals you set for yourself in chapters 11 and 12 have a direct impact on any weight-loss desires you may have. For those who are uniquely motivated to work on attaining a healthy body weight, I encourage you to write down a goal that is important to you. It should include how much weight you want to lose, how many weeks you will strive to reduce your calories, and the details of your exercise plans. Write your goal down here.

My Weight Loss Goal

I will lose _____ pounds.

I will focus on healthy foods and reduce my calories every day for _____ weeks.

My exercise plan is (detailed): _____

_____

_____

_____

To demonstrate how committed you are, share this goal with someone, sign it, and have the other person sign it as a witness.

Signature:_____ Date:_____

Signature:_____ Date:_____

POINTS TO REMEMBER

- Weight loss and healthy weight maintenance are side effects of a healthy lifestyle. Adopt a healthy lifestyle and you will be more likely to have a healthy weight.

- American culture and aggressive food marketing make attaining a healthy weight hard to do. You must control the size of your food portions and the amount of food you eat. Don't leave this job to the food industry.

- Good nutrition and physical activity behaviors are the keys to healthy weight. Stop the healthy behaviors and your weight will return to prior levels.

- Learn wisdom from the wise; live like the weight-control masters.

- Low-carbohydrate diets, as well as other kinds of diets, can help you reduce the number of calories you eat, but don't go on a diet just to later go off a diet. Change your lifestyle.

- Recognize the triggers that make you want to eat and plan ways to deal with those triggers.

BEHAVIOR CHANGE ▶

MEDICATIONS ▶

GOOD NUTRITION ▶

PHYSICAL ACTIVITY ▶

HEALTHY EMPLOYEES ▶

INSURANCE PREMIUMS ▶

SCHOOLS ▶

RESTAURANTS ▶

CHAPTER / 14

The Winds of Change

They must often change who would be
constant in happiness or wisdom.
—Confucius (551 BC–479 BC)

I N THE UNITED STATES, A CULTURAL CHANGE HAS BEGUN. The number
of individuals who are openly concerned about health and quality of
life has grown. They are now a force so strong that they are beginning
to force environmental and societal changes. Pick up any newspaper from
any city in the country and you will see articles about weight control,
nutrition, and physical activity—all part of a healthy lifestyle. Interest
from the media has also grown dramatically. Interest from the medical
community grows every day; medical journals such as the *New England
Journal of Medicine* and the *Journal of the American Medical Association*
now regularly publish research findings from studies on the effects of good
nutrition and physical activity. Historically, these journals rarely published
studies on these topics.

The cultural change in attitudes about health has resulted in changes
in how we treat chronic-disease risk factors as well. Just a few years ago
the standard treatment for high blood cholesterol was medication. Now
standard treatment begins with lots of TLC (therapeutic lifestyle change)—
a medical way to say "start living a healthy lifestyle."[1] In the near future,

standard treatment of high blood pressure is also likely to start with some TLC.[2] Medical advice to start living a healthy lifestyle is not going to be just for those who have major health risks. This advice is also appropriate for people who are overweight or who have any chronic-disease risk factors that are even slightly above normal.[3]

These initial changes in the treatment and prevention of chronic diseases are just one example of how the future of medicine will most likely include prescriptions for a strong dose of healthy behaviors. After successful behavior change, if health risks are still too high, medications should be prescribed.

Momentum for these changes is even working its way through the federal government. Now more than ever, the federal government is increasing its support for the promotion of healthy lifestyles. The Centers for Disease Control and Prevention recently put out a notice seeking applications from scientists doing health-promotion research. It was the first notice for health-promotion research the CDC had done in many years, and they received five times the number of applications they had anticipated.[4]

The U.S. Department of Health and Human Services (HHS) has made disease prevention and healthy living a priority and is starting many different programs designed to help the public live a healthy lifestyle. Many of these can be found at the HHS Web site, www.healthierus.gov. The U.S. Department of Agriculture is planning to update the Food Guide Pyramid. The update will be based on the same scientific information presented in chapters 5, 6, 7, and 8 of this book. You already have the information.

A healthy employee is more productive and doesn't require as much health care. A healthy employee is happier and actually saves the company money. A healthy employee is one who lives a healthy lifestyle.

Your Employer Is Changing

The average cost of providing health care for a family is at least $9,068 per year[5]; that is a lot of money. Since we don't have to pay that much directly out of our salaries, we don't feel the total financial burden each month when we get paid, but every American is still paying. The money to fund health care comes from the higher price you pay for goods and services, from your taxes, and from your employer's contributions. And each year, workers and employers pay more for health insurance. In 2003, for example, health care costs for companies across the United States increased 14% on average; in the western United States, the increase was 16%.[5]

What does this have to do with a healthy lifestyle? Many companies have discovered that the total cost of health care for their employees is directly related to the health of their employees. In other words, employers who actively help their employees stay healthy get better employees and save money. A healthy employee is more productive and doesn't require as much health care. A healthy employee is happier and actually saves the company money. A healthy employee is one who lives a healthy lifestyle.

To help employees adopt healthy lifestyles, many companies (both large and small) offer their employees access to programs designed to promote healthy living. The number of worksites that offer health-promotion programs increases every year as companies face higher and higher health care costs for their employees.[6,7] Why should you care if your employer has a health-promotion program? If you work at one of these places, you have access to a fantastic support group and a health-promotion team. Your worksite can help you achieve your healthy lifestyle goals. Worksite health-promotion programs provide fun, effective programs to help you change eating habits and physical activity behaviors.

Your Insurance Is Changing

If you apply for life insurance and you smoke, you can still get a life insurance policy, but because you smoke, it is going to cost you more. Smoking is no longer the only reason why both life and health insurance premiums increase. More and more insurance companies are "risk rating" their insurance. That means if you are obese or physically inactive, for example, you may have to pay more for insurance. Insurance companies know all about healthy lifestyles; they prefer to insure healthy people, and more companies are now basing some premiums on health risks and whether or not a person has a healthy lifestyle.

Schools Are Changing

Pressure from parents, physicians, school health nurses, and a few health-conscious teachers is slowly improving school environments. Many schools have recently adopted new policies regarding vending machines. In 2003, California became the first state to ban soft drink sales at elementary and junior high schools. About two dozen states are considering limits or even total bans on vending machine products, while about 20 states already restrict students' access to junk food until after lunch. Still other schools are trying to keep everyone happy by requiring vendors to make 70% of the food offerings healthy. Soda machines are offering more water, low-fat milk, 100% fruit juices, and low-calorie sports drinks.

Many state departments of education are implementing or revisiting the idea of mandatory physical education for children from kindergarten through high school. If children can learn to be physically active when they are young, they may carry these skills and habits into adulthood.

Your Food and Physical Activity Environment Is Changing

McDonald's announced in 2002 that it was going to introduce a new cooking oil in its restaurants that contained half the amount of trans fats as the previous frying oil. After two years, the only thing that has changed is McDonald's legal standing. A lawsuit has been filed against McDonald's because they made that big announcement but then never made any changes. Lawsuits are one way to force change. As soon as one fast food restaurant finally stops frying in trans fats, others will follow. No restaurant has taken the lead so far, but it is only a matter of time before change sweeps the industry. In the future, trans fats will most likely be removed completely from the food supply. More restaurants now offer healthier choices on their menus, with many fast food restaurants marketing sandwiches on whole wheat bread and a variety of salads.

Cities and counties are developing trails and bike paths. Airlines are offering exercise opportunities at airports and even in flight. Churches are using church facilities and community centers to teach their members about healthy lifestyles. Some churches encourage members to bring only healthy foods to church socials and dinners. There is a subtle breeze blowing through communities that hints at the need to replace unhealthy behaviors with healthy ones.

Science Is Changing

Almost every day, scientific journals publish new research on healthy living. The only reason we know good food and exercise are important is because of studies that have shown the benefits of such healthy lifestyle choices. Many of these articles are picked up by the media, and you read about the studies in the press. Several newsletters have been created to inform the public about advances in healthy living. I suggest the Berkeley Wellness Letter (www.berkeleywellness.com), the Mayo Clinic Health

Letter (www.mayoclinic.com), and the Harvard Health Letter (www.
health.harvard.edu/hhp/home.do). These are accurate, unbiased sources
of new health information. Working adults might like the Well Workplace
Newsletter (www.welcoa.org). If you are ambitious, you can go to the
Web site of the National Library of Congress at www.pubmed.gov, type in
"lifestyle," and see just about every scientific article in the world on this
subject. This is where the science can be seen the way it was first presented
by the researchers who conducted the studies. This is the science that is
slowly changing the world.

Best of All, You Are Changing

If you have been patient enough to read everything to this point, you
understand how lifestyle can be both the culprit behind and the cure of
America's poor health. You realize that you have the skills and knowledge to
change, just like Joe, who said this in an e-mail message he sent me:

> Last year I decided to get serious about my health. Type two diabetes
> is prevalent in my family and my blood pressure was high (150 over
> 85). Over the last year I have lost 105 pounds and my blood pressure
> and pulse are perfect. I am now down to 205 lbs. and my blood
> pressure is 112 over 50 with a resting pulse of 53. My wife and I have
> been working on this together and she has lost 60 pounds herself. We
> exercise together every morning and have changed the way we eat.
> This new lifestyle has transformed my life.
>
> Joe
> St. Louis, Missouri

That reads like an infomercial! I didn't go to his house and take mea-
surements to verify if what he said was true. I don't have to. I get letters all
the time from people who want to tell someone about their successes. I love
hearing about the changes people experience. I don't think very many people can change as much as Joe and his wife; his story is not typical unless
you are as motivated as he was—people like Joe can probably make changes
without help from anyone. But change is the common theme among everyone who writes, and change is the main reason why I wrote this book.

It is my most sincere hope that the information I have presented here
helps you understand what many health professionals already know—a
healthy lifestyle is the key to a long, high-quality life. Healthy lifestyle choices
and changes are not going to solve all of America's health problems, but they
will have a greater impact on your life than anything else you can do.

Tell me about it!

As you improve your lifestyle and start to experience change, I want to know about it. Here is my e-mail address: letters@theculpritandthecure.com. Write me. I promise to read it. Tell me about any successes or failures you have as you try to adopt a new lifestyle. I promise to keep your e-mail address confidential. You can also leave me comments on the Web site: www.theculpritandthecure.com.

POINTS TO REMEMBER

- Share this book with someone you really care about.

- Enough points to remember! Get out there and get started!

References

Chapter 1

1. The Harvard Report on Cancer Prevention. Causes of human cancer. *Cancer Causes and Control.* 1996:7(1)S7–S9.

2. Block, G, Patterson B, and Subar A. Fruit, vegetables, and cancer prevention: A review of epidemiological evidence. *Nutr and Cancer.* 1992; 18:1–29.

3. Behavioral Risk Factor Surveillance System, Centers for Disease Control, 2002. www.cdc.gov/brfss

4. Behavioral Risk Factor Surveillance System, Centers for Disease Control, 2001. www.cdc.gov/brfss

5. Stampfer MJ, Hu FB, Manson JE, Rimm EB, Willett WC. Primary prevention of coronary heart disease in women through diet and lifestyle. *N Engl J Med.* 2000 Jul 6;343(1):16–22.

6. Platz EA, Willett WC, Colditz GA, Rimm EB, Spiegelman D, Giovannucci E. Proportion of colon cancer risk that might be preventable in a cohort of middle-aged US men. *Cancer Causes Control.* 2000 Aug;11(7):579–88.

7. Hu FB, Manson JE, Stampfer MJ, Colditz G, Liu S, Solomon CG, Willett WC. Diet, lifestyle, and the risk of type 2 diabetes mellitus in women. *N Engl J Med.* 2001 Sep 13;345(11):790–7.

8. Fraser GE, Shavlik DJ. Ten years of life: Is it a matter of choice? *Arch Intern Med.* 2001 Jul 9;161(13):1645–52.

9. Fontaine KR, Redden DT, Wang C, Westfall AO, Allison DB. Years of life lost due to obesity. *JAMA.* 2003 Jan 8;289(2):187–93.

10. Enstrom JE. Health practices and cancer mortality among active California Mormons. *J Natl Cancer Inst.* 1989 Dec 6;81(23):1807–14.

11. Winkelmann BR, Hager J, Kraus WE, Merlini P, Keavney B, Grant PJ, Muhlestein JB,Granger CB. Genetics of coronary heart disease: current knowledge and research principles. *Am Heart J.* 2000 Oct;140(4):S11–26.

12. Lubitz J, Cai L, Kramarow E, Lentzner H. Health, Life Expectancy, and Health Care Spending among the Elderly. *N Engl J Med.* 2003 Sep 11;349(11):1048–1055.

13. Fries JF. Successful aging—an emerging paradigm of gerontology. *Clin Geriatr Med.* 2002 Aug;18(3):371–82.

14. Wang BW, Ramey DR, Schettler JD, Hubert HB, Fries JF. Postponed development of disability in elderly runners: a 13-year longitudinal study. *Arch Intern Med.* 2002 Nov 11;162(20):2285–94.

15. Hubert HB, Bloch DA, Oehlert JW, Fries JF. Lifestyle habits and compression of morbidity. *J Gerontol A Biol Sci Med Sci.* 2002 Jun;57(6): M347–51.

16. Fries JF. Aging, cumulative disability, and the compression of morbidity. *Compr Ther.* 2001 Winter;27(4):322–9.

17. Esselstyn CB Jr. Resolving the Coronary Artery Disease Epidemic Through Plant-Based Nutrition. *Prev Cardiol.* 2001 Autumn;4(4):171–177.

18. Esselstyn CB Jr. Updating a 12-year experience with arrest and reversal therapy for coronary heart disease (an overdue requiem for palliative cardiology). *Am J Cardiol.* 1999 Aug 1;84(3):339–41, A8.

19. Ornish D, Scherwitz LW, Billings JH, Brown SE, Gould KL, Merritt TA, Sparler S, Armstrong WT, Ports TA, Kirkeeide RL, Hogeboom C, Brand RJ. Intensive lifestyle changes for reversal of coronary heart disease. *JAMA.* 1998 Dec 16;280(23):2001–7.

20. Gould KL, Ornish D, Scherwitz L, Brown S, Edens RP, Hess MJ, Mullani N, Bolomey L, Dobbs F, Armstrong WT, et al. Changes in myocardial perfusion abnormalities by positron emission tomography after long-term, intense

---

risk factor modification. *JAMA.* 1995 Sep 20;274(11):894–901.

21. Diabetes Prevention Program Research Group. Within-trial cost-effectiveness of lifestyle intervention or metformin for the primary prevention of type 2 diabetes. *Diabetes Care.* 2003 Sep;26(9):2518–23.

22. Knowler WC, Barrett-Connor E, Fowler SE, Hamman RF, Lachin JM, Walker EA, Nathan DM; Diabetes Prevention Program Research Group. Reduction in the incidence of type 2 diabetes with lifestyle intervention or Metformin. *N Engl J Med.* 2002 Feb 7;346(6):393–403.

23. Aldana SG, Greenlaw R, Diehl HA, Englert H, Jackson R. Impact of the coronary health improvement project (CHIP) on several employee populations. *J Occup Environ Med.* 2002 Sep;44(9):831–9.

24. Surgeon Generals' Report on Physical Activity and Health, 1996, www.cdc.gov/nccdphp/sgr/sgr.htm

25. Willett WC, Stampfer MJ. Rebuilding the food pyramid. *Sci Am.* 2003 Jan; 288(1):64–71.

26. CDC, National Center for Health Statistics, National Health and Nutrition Examination Survey. Health, United States (Table 70) 2002.

27. Brown Bread Versus White, *British Medical Journal.* 1937:ii:752.

28. Liu S. Whole-grain foods, dietary fiber, and type 2 diabetes: searching for a kernel of truth. *Am J Clin Nutr.* 2003 Mar;77(3):527–9.

29. Andersen RE, Crespo CJ, Bartlett SJ, Cheskin LJ, Pratt M. Relationship of physical activity and television watching with body weight and level of fatness among children: results from the Third National Health and Nutrition Examination Survey. *JAMA.* 1998 Mar 25;279(12):938–42.

30. Nestle, M. Food Politics: How the food industry influences nutrition and health, 2002, University of California Press, Berkeley California.

31. Ministry of Agriculture, Fisheries, and Food. Household food consumption and expenditure, 1990. With a study of trends over the period, 1940–1990. Annual Report of the National Food Survey Committee. London: Her Majesty's Stationary Office, 1991.

32. Employee Benefit Research Institute, Adequacy of Retirement Income Remains a Policy Concern, May 20, 2002. www.ebri.org

33. Jacobs, Francine. *Breakthrough: The True Story of Penicillin.* New York: Dodd, Mead & Company, 1985.

Chapter 2

1. National Vital Statistics Report, Vol. 50, No. 16, page 8, September 16, 2002.

2. Menotti A, Keys A, Kromhout D, Blackburn H, Aravanis C, Bloemberg B, Buzina R,Dontas A, Fidanza F, Giampaoli S, et al. Inter-cohort differences in coronary heart disease mortality

in the 25-year follow-up of the seven countries study. *Eur J Epidemiol.* 1993 Sep;9(5):527–36.

3. Antunes JL, Toporcov TN, De Andrade FP. Trends and patterns of cancer mortality in European countries. *Eur J Cancer Prev.* 2003 Oct;12(5):367–72.

4. Framingham Heart Study 2003, found on the Web at http://www.framingham.com/heart/

5. Friedenreich CM. Physical activity and cancer prevention: from observational to intervention research. *Cancer Epidemiol Biomarkers Prev.* 2001 Apr;10(4):287–301.

6. Clare DA, Catignani GL, Swaisgood HE. Biodefense properties of milk: the role of antimicrobial proteins and peptides. *Curr Pharm Des.* 2003;9(16):1239–55.

7. Miller GD, Jarvis JK, McBean LD. The importance of meeting calcium needs with foods. *J Am Coll Nutr.* 2001 Apr;20(2 Suppl):168S–185S.

8. Enstrom JE. Health practices and cancer mortality among active California Mormons. *J Natl Cancer Inst.* 1989 Dec 6;81(23):1807–14.

9. Willett W. Lessons from dietary studies in Adventists and questions for the future. *Am J Clin Nutr.* 2003 Sep;78(3 Suppl):539S–543S.

Chapter 3

1. U.S. National Center for Health Statistics, National Vital Statistics Report, vol. 51, no. 5, March 14, 2003. Web: www.cdc.gov/nchs.

2. Enos WF, Holmes RH, Beyer J. Coronary disease among United States soldiers killed in action in Korea: preliminary report. *JAMA.* 1953;152:1090–1093.

3. Joseph A, Ackerman D, Talley JD, Johnstone J, Kupersmith J. Manifestations of coronary atherosclerosis in young trauma victims—an autopsy study. *J Am Coll Cardiol.* 1993 Aug;22(2):459–67.

4. Raitakari OT, et al. Cardiovascular risk factors in childhood and carotid artery intima-media thickness in adulthood: the Cardiovascular Risk in Young Finns Study. *JAMA.* 2003 Nov 5;290(17):2277–83.

5. Tuzcu EM, Kapadia SR, Tutar E, Ziada KM, Hobbs RE, McCarthy PM, Young JB, Nissen SE. High prevalence of coronary atherosclerosis in asymptomatic teenagers and young adults: evidence from intravascular ultrasound. *Circulation.* 2001 Jun 5; 103(22): 2705–10.

6. Knoflach M, et al. Cardiovascular risk factors and atherosclerosis in young males: ARMY study (Atherosclerosis Risk-Factors in Male Youngsters). *Circulation.* 2003 Sep 2;108(9):1064–9.

7. Murata M. Secular trends in growth and changes in eating patterns of Japanese children. *Am J Clin Nutr.* 2000: 72(Suppl. 5):1379S–1383S.

8. Kitamura A, Iso H, Iida M, Naito Y, Sato S, Jacobs DR, Nakamura M, Shimamoto T,

Komachi Y. Trends in the incidence of coronary heart disease and stroke and the prevalence of cardiovascular risk factors among Japanese men from 1963 to 1994. *Am J Med*. 2002 Feb 1; 112(2): 104–9.

9. Robertson TL, Kato H, Rhoads GG, Kagan A, Marmot M, Syme SL, Gordon T, Worth RM, Belsky JL, Dock DS, Miyanishi M, Kawamoto S. Epidemiologic studies of coronary heart disease and stroke in Japanese men living in Japan, Hawaii and California. Incidence of myocardial infarction and death from coronary heart disease. *Am J Cardiol*. 1977 Feb; 39(2): 239–43.

10. Guerra A, Feldl F, Kolezko B. Fatty acid composition of plasma lipids in healthy Portugues children: is the Mediterranean diet disappearing? *Ann Nutr Metab*. 2001: 45:78–81.

11. Zheng et al. Sudden cardiac death in U.S. young adults, 1989–96, *Circulation*. 2001;103:1345.

12. Gould KL, Ornish D, Kirkeeide R, Brown S, Stuart Y, Buchi M, Billings J, Armstrong W, Ports T, Scherwitz L. Improved stenosis geometry by quantitative coronary arteriography after vigorous risk factor modification. *Am J Cardiol*. 1992, 69, 845–853.

13. Gould KL, Ornish D, Scherwitz L, Brown S, Edens RP, Hess MJ, Mullani N, Bolomey L, Dobbs F, & Armstrong WT, et al. Changes in myocardial perfusion abnormalities by positron emission tomography after long-term intense risk factor modification. *JAMA*. 1995,274,(11), 894–901.

14. Ornish D, Brown SE, Scherwitz LW, Billings JH, Armstrong WT, Ports TA, McLanahan SM, Kirkeeide RL, Brand RJ, & Gould KL. Can lifestyle changes reverse coronary heart disease? The Lifestyle Heart Trial. *Lancet*. 1990, 336, 129–133.

15. Li S, et al. Childhood cardiovascular risk factors and carotid vascular changes in adulthood: the Bogalusa Heart Study. *JAMA*. 2003 Nov 5;290(17):2271–6.

16. Berenson GS. Childhood risk factors predict adult risk associated with subclinical cardiovascular disease. The Bogalusa Heart Study. *Am J Cardiol*. 2002 Nov 21; 90(10C): 3L–7L.

17. Davis PH, Dawson JD, Riley WA, Lauer RM. Carotid intimal-medial thickness is related to cardiovascular risk factors measured from childhood through middle age: The Muscatine Study. *Circulation*. 2001 Dec 4; 104(23): 2815–9.

18. Urbina EM, Srinivasan SR, Tang R, Bond MG, Kieltyka L, Berenson GS. Impact of multiple coronary risk factors on the intima-media thickness of different segments of carotid artery in healthy young adults (The Bogalusa Heart Study). *Am J Cardiol*. 2002 Nov 1; 90(9): 953–8.

19. Stary C. Lipid and macrophage accumulations in arteries of children and development of atherosclerosis. *Am J Clin Nutr*. 2000; 72 (Suppl. 5):1297S–1306S.

20. McGill Jr HC, McMahan CA, Herderick EE, et al., for the PDAY Research Group. Effects of coronary heart disease risk factors on atherosclerosis of selected regions of the aorta and right coronary artery. *Arterioscler Thromb Vasc Biol*. 2000; 20:836–845.

21. Sorensen KE, Celermajer DS, Georgakopoulos D, et al. Impairment of endothelium-dependent dilation is an early event in children with familial hypercholesterolemia and is related to the lipoprotein(a) level. *J Clin Invest*. 1994; 93:50–55.

22. Aggoun Y, Bonnet D, Sidi D, et al. Arterial mechanical changes in children with familial hypercholesterolemia. *Arterioscler Thromb Vasc Biol*. 2000; 20:2070–2075.

23. Leeson CP, Whincup PH, Cook DG, et al. Cholesterol and arterial distensibility in the first decade of life: a population-based study. *Circulation*. 2000; 101:1533–1538.

24. Napoli C, D'Armiento FP, Mancini FP, et al. Fatty streak formation occurs in human fetal aortas and is greatly enhanced by maternal hypercholesterolemia. Intimal accumulation of low density lipoprotein and its oxidation precede monocyte recruitment into early atherosclerotic lesions. *J Clin Invest*. 1997; 100:2680–2690.

25. Behavioral Risk Factor Surveillance System, Centers for Disease Control, 2002. www.cdc.gov/brfss

26. Block G, Patterson B, and Subar A. Fruit, vegetables, and cancer prevention: A review of epidemiological evidence. *Nutr and Cancer*. 1992; 18:1–29.

27. CDC. Annual smoking-attributable mortality, years of potential life lost, and economic costs— United States, 1995–1999. *MMWR* 2002;51: 300–3. Also available on the Web at http://www. cdc.gov/mmwr/preview/mmwrhtml/mm5114a2. htm

28. U.S. Department of Commerce, Health Insurance Coverage in the United States: 2003, also available on the Web at http://www.census. gov/prod/2003pubs/p60-223.pdf

29. Collins TC, Petersen NJ, Suarez-Almazor M. The prevalence of peripheral arterial disease in a racially diverse population. *Arch Intern Med*. 2003 Jun 23; 163(12): 1469–74.

30. Bourassa MG. Long-term vein graft patency. *Curr Opin Cardiol*. 1994; 9:685–691.

31. Hirshfeld JW Jr, Schwartz JS, Jugo R, MacDonald RG, Goldberg S, Savage MP, Bass TA, Vetrovec G, Cowley M, Taussig AS, et al. Restenosis after coronary angioplasty: a multivariate statistical model to relate lesion and procedure variables to restenosis. The M-HEART Investigators. *J Am Coll Cardiol*. 1991 Sep; 18(3): 647–56.

32. Bauters C, Isner JM. The biology of restenosis. In: Topol EJ, ed. *Textbook of Cardiovascular Medicine*. Philadelphia, Pennsylvania: Lippincott-Raven; 1998:2465–2490.

33. Rajagopal V, Rockson SG. Coronary restenosis: a review of mechanisms and management. *Am J Med*. 2003 Nov; 115(7): 547–53.

34. Galuska DA, Will JC, Serdula MK, Ford ES. Are health care professionals advising obese patients to lose weight? *JAMA*. 1999 Oct 27;282(16):1581–2.

35. Wee CC, McCarthy EP, Davis RB, Phillips RS. Physician counseling about exercise. *JAMA*. 1999 Oct 27;282(16):1581–2.

36. Haynes RB, McDonald HP, Garg AX. Helping patients follow prescribed treatment: clinical applications. *JAMA*. 2002 Dec 11; 288(22):2880–3.

Chapter 4

1. Stampfer MJ, Hu FB, Manson JE, Rimm EB, Willett WC. Primary prevention of coronary heart disease in women through diet and lifestyle. *N Engl J Med*. 2000 Jul 6;343(1):16–22.

2. Framingham Heart Study 2003, found on the Web at http://www.framingham.com/heart/

3. Chobanian AV, Bakris GL, Black HR, Cushman WC, Green LA, Izzo JL Jr, Jones DW, Materson BJ, Oparil S, Wright JT Jr, Roccella EJ; National Heart, Lung, and Blood Institute Joint National Committee on Prevention, Detection, Evaluation, and Treatment of High Blood Pressure; National High Blood Pressure Education Program Coordinating Committee. The Seventh Report of the Joint National Committee on Prevention, Detection, Evaluation, and Treatment of High Blood Pressure: the JNC 7 report. *JAMA*. 2003 May 21;289(19):2560-72.

4. Third Report of the National Cholesterol Education Program (NCEP) Expert Panel on Detection, Evaluation, and Treatment of High Blood Cholesterol in Adults (Adult Treatment Panel III) National Cholesterol Education Program, National Heart, Lung, and Blood Institute, National Institutes of Health, NIH Publication No. 01-3670, May 2001

5. www.nhlbi.nih.gov/health/public/heart/obesity/lose_wt/bmi_dis.htm

6. Aldana SG, Greenlaw R, Diehl HA, Englert H, Jackson R. Impact of the Coronary Health Improvement Project (CHIP) on several employee populations. *J Occup Environ Med*. 2002;44(9)36-45.

7. Aldana S, Greenlaw R, Diehl H, Salberg A, Merrill R, Ohmine S, Thomas C, Olsen J. The effects of an intensive lifestyle modification program, *J Am Diet Assoc*. (in press).

8. Manson JE, Tosteson H, Ridker PM, Satterfield S, Hebert P, O'Connor GT, Buring JE, Hennekens CH. The primary prevention of myocardial infarction. *N Engl J Med*. 1992;326:1406-14.

9. Blair SN, Kohl HW, Paffenbarger RS, Clark DG, Cooper KH, and Gibbons LW. Physical fitness and all cause mortality: A prospective study of health men and women. *JAMA*. 262:2395-2401, 1989.

10. U.S. Department of Health and Human Services, Physical Activity and Health: A Report of the Surgeon General. Centers for Disease Control and Prevention, National Center for Chronic Disease Prevention and Health Promotion, The President's Council on Physical Fitness and Sports. Atlanta, GA, (1996). Found on the Web at www.cdc.gov/nccdphp/sgr/ataglan.htm

11. Food, Nutrition, and the Prevention of Cancer: A Global Perspective, World Cancer Research Fund, American Institute for Cancer Research, 1997. Found on the Web at http://www.wcrf.org/report/index.lasso

12. Cook S, Weitzman M, Auinger P, Nguyen M, Dietz WH. Prevalence of a metabolic syndrome phenotype in adolescents: findings from the third National Health and Nutrition Examination Survey, 1988-1994. *Arch Pediatr Adolesc Med*. 2003 Aug;157(8):821-7.

13. Ford ES, Giles WH, Dietz WH. Prevalence of the metabolic syndrome among US adults: findings from the third National Health and Nutrition Examination Survey. *JAMA*. 2002 Jan 16;287(3):356-9.

14. Park YW, Zhu S, Palaniappan L, Heshka S, Carnethon MR, Heymsfield SB. The metabolic syndrome: prevalence and associated risk factor findings in the US population from the Third National Health and Nutrition Examination Survey, 1988-1994. *Arch Intern Med*. 2003 Feb 24;163(4):427-36.

15. Peeters A, Barendregt JJ, Willekens F, Mackenbach JP, Al Mamun A, Bonneux L; NEDCOM, the Netherlands Epidemiology and Demography Compression of Morbidity Research Group. Obesity in adulthood and its consequences for life expectancy: a life-table analysis. *Ann Intern Med*. 2003 Jan 7;138(1):24-32.

16. CDC, National Center for Health Statistics, National Health and Nutrition Examination Survey. Health, United States (Table 70) 2002.

17. Flegal KM, Carroll MD, Ogden CL, Johnson CL. Prevalence and trends in obesity among US adults, 1999-2000. *JAMA*. 2002 Oct 9;288(14):1723-7.

18. Ogden CL, Flegal KM, Carroll MD, Johnson CL. Prevalence and trends in overweight among US children and adolescents, 1999-2000. *JAMA*. 2002 Oct 9;288(14):1728-32.

19. Behavioral Risk Factor Surveillance System, Centers for Disease Control, 2001 www.cdc.gov/brfss

20. Ham S, Yore M, Fulton J, Kohl III H, Prevalence of No Leisure-Time Physical Activity—35 States and the District of Columbia, 1988—2002, *MMWR,* February 6, 2004 / 53(04);82-86. Found on the Web at: http://www.cdc.gov/mmwr/preview/mmwrhtml/mm5304a4.htm

21. Wright J, Kennedy-Stephenson J, Wang C, McDowell M, Johnson C, Trends in Intake of Energy and Macronutrients—United States, 1971—2000, *MMWR,* February 6, 2004 / 53(04);80-82. Found on the Web at: http://www.cdc.gov/mmwr/preview/mmwrhtml/mm5304a3.htm

22. Kim S, Symons M, Popkin BM. Contrasting socioeconomic profiles related to healthier lifestyles in China and the United States. *Am J Epidemiol.* 2004 Jan 15;159(2):184-91.

23. Witteman JC, Willett WC, Stampfer MJ, Colditz GA, Sacks FM, Speizer FE, Rosner B, Hennekens CH. A prospective study of nutritional factors and hypertension among US women. *Circulation.* 1989 Nov;80(5):1320-7.

24. Denke MA, Sempos CT, Grundy SM. Excess body weight. An underrecognized contributor to high blood cholesterol levels in white American men. *Arch Intern Med.* 1993 10;153(9):1093-103.

25. Manson JE, Colditz GA, Stampfer MJ, Willett WC, Rosner B, Monson RR, Speizer FE, Hennekens CH. A prospective study of obesity and risk of coronary heart disease in women. *N Engl J Med.* 1990 Mar 29;322(13):882-9.

26. Rimm EB, Stampfer MJ, Giovannucci E, Ascherio A, Spiegelman D, Colditz GA,Willett WC. Body size and fat distribution as predictors of coronary heart disease among middle-aged and older US men. *Am J Epidemiol.* 1995 Jun 15;141(12):1117-27.

27. Rexrode KM, Hennekens CH, Willett WC, Colditz GA, Stampfer MJ, Rich-Edwards JW, Speizer FE, Manson JE. A prospective study of body mass index, weight change, and risk of stroke in women. *JAMA.* 1997 May 21;277(19):1539-45.

28. Folsom AR, Kaye SA, Sellers TA, Hong CP, Cerhan JR, Potter JD, Prineas RJ. Body fat distribution and 5-year risk of death in older women. *JAMA.* 1993 Jan 27;269(4):483-7.

29. Abu-Abid S, Szold A, Klausner J. Obesity and cancer. *J Med.* 2002;33(1-4):73-86.

30. Van Itallie TB. Health implications of overweight and obesity in the United States. *Ann Intern Med.* 1985 Dec;103(6 (Pt 2)):983-8.

31. Ballard-Barbash R, Swanson CA. Body weight: estimation of risk for breast and endometrial cancers. *Am J Clin Nutr.* 1996 Mar;63(3 Suppl):437S-41S.

32. Stampfer MJ, Maclure KM, Colditz GA, Manson JE, Willett WC. Risk of symptomatic gallstones in women with severe obesity. *Am J Clin Nutr.* 1992 Mar;55(3):652-8.

33. Maclure KM, Hayes KC, Colditz GA, Stampfer MJ, Speizer FE, Willett WC. Weight, diet, and the risk of symptomatic gallstones in middle-aged women. *N Engl J Med.* 1989 Aug 31;321(9):563-9.

34. Camargo CA Jr, Weiss ST, Zhang S, Willett WC, Speizer FE. Prospective study of body mass index, weight change, and risk of adult-onset asthma in women. *Arch Intern Med.* 1999 Nov 22;159(21):2582-8.

35. Gustafson D, Rothenberg E, Blennow K, Steen B, Skoog I. An 18-year follow-up of overweight and risk of Alzheimer's disease. *Arch Intern Med.* 2003 Jul 14;163(13):1524-8.

36. Manson JE, Colditz GA, Stampfer MJ, Willett WC, Krolewski AS, Rosner B, Arky RA, Speizer FE, Hennekens CH. A prospective study of maturity-onset diabetes mellitus and risk of coronary heart disease and stroke in women. *Arch Intern Med.* 1991 Jun;151(6):1141-7.

37. Chan JM, Rimm EB, Colditz GA, Stampfer MJ, Willett WC. Obesity, fat distribution, and weight gain as risk factors for clinical diabetes in men. *Diabetes Care.* 1994 Sep;17(9):961-9.

38. Kaye SA, Folsom AR, Sprafka JM, Prineas RJ, Wallace RB. Increased incidence of diabetes mellitus in relation to abdominal adiposity in older women. *J Clin Epidemiol.* 1991;44(3):329-34.

39. Narayan KM, Boyle JP, Thompson TJ, Sorensen SW, Williamson DF. Lifetime risk for diabetes mellitus in the United States. *JAMA.* 2003 Oct 8;290(14):1884-90.

40. Knowler WC, Barrett-Connor E, Fowler SE, Hamman RF, Lachin JM, Walker EA, Nathan DM; Diabetes Prevention Program Research Group. Reduction in the incidence of type 2 diabetes with lifestyle intervention or metformin. *N Engl J Med.* 2002 Feb 7;346(6):393-403.

41. Tuomilehto J, Lindstrom J, Eriksson JG, Valle TT, Hamalainen H, Ilanne-Parikka P, Keinanen-Kiukaanniemi S, Laakso M, Louheranta A, Rastas M, Salminen V, Uusitupa M; Finnish Diabetes Prevention Study Group. Prevention of type 2 diabetes mellitus by changes in lifestyle among subjects with impaired glucose tolerance. *N Engl J Med.* 2001 May 3;344(18):1343-50.

42. Case CC, Jones PH, Nelson K, O'Brian Smith E, Ballantyne CM. Impact of weight loss on the metabolic syndrome. *Diabetes Obes Metab.* 2002 Nov;4(6):407-14.

43. Gregg EW, Gerzoff RB, Caspersen CJ, Williamson DF, Narayan KM. Relationship of walking to mortality among US adults with diabetes. *Arch Intern Med.* 2003 Jun 23;163(12):1440-7.

Chapter 5

1. Adams JF, Enstrom A. Dietary intake of whole grain vs. recommendations. *Cereal Foods World,* 2000;45:75–78.

2. Slavin J. Why whole grains are protective: biological mechanisms. *Proc Nutr Soc.* 2003 Feb;62(1):129–34.

3. Slavin JL, Jacobs D, Marquart L, Wiemer K. The role of whole grains in disease prevention. *J Am Diet Assoc.* 2001 Jul;101(7):780–5.

4. Pereira MA, O'Reilly E, Augustsson K, Fraser GE, Goldbourt U, Heitmann BL, Hallmans G, Knekt P, Liu S, Pietinen P, Spiegelman D, Stevens J, Virtamo J, Willett WC, Ascherio A. Dietary fiber and risk of coronary heart disease: a pooled analysis of cohort studies. *Arch Intern Med.* 2004 Feb 23;164(4):370–6.

5. Pereira MA, Pins JJ. Dietary fiber and cardiovascular disease: experimental and epidemiologic advances. *Curr Atheroscler Rep.* 2000 Nov;2(6):494–502.

6. Liu S, Stampfer MJ, Hu FB, Giovannucci E, Rimm E, Manson JE, Hennekens CH, Willett WC. Whole-grain consumption and risk of coronary heart disease: results from the Nurses' Health Study. *Am J Clin Nutr.* 1999 Sep;70(3):412–9.

7. Jacobs DR Jr, Marquart L, Slavin J, Kushi LH. Whole-grain intake and cancer: an expanded review and meta-analysis. *Nutr Cancer.* 1998;30(2):85–96.

8. Jang Y, Lee JH, Kim OY, Park HY, Lee SY. Consumption of whole grain and legume powder reduces insulin demand, lipid peroxidation, and plasma homocysteine concentrations in patients with coronary artery disease: randomized controlled clinical trial. *Arterioscler Thromb Vasc Biol.* 2001 Dec;21(12):2065–71.

9. Liu S. Intake of refined carbohydrates and whole grain foods in relation to risk of type 2 diabetes mellitus and coronary heart disease. *J Am Coll Nutr.* 2002 Aug;21(4):298–306.

10. Liu S, Manson JE, Stampfer MJ, Hu FB, Giovannucci E, Colditz GA, Hennekens CH, Willett WC. A prospective study of whole-grain intake and risk of type 2 diabetes mellitus in US women. *Am J Public Health.* 2000 Sep;90(9):1409–15.

11. Fung TT, Hu FB, Pereira MA, Liu S, Stampfer MJ, Colditz GA, Willett WC. Whole-grain intake and the risk of type 2 diabetes: a prospective study in men. *Am J Clin Nutr.* 2002 Sep;76(3):535–40.

12. Liu S, Manson JE, Stampfer MJ, Rexrode KM, Hu FB, Rimm EB, Willett WC. Whole grain consumption and risk of ischemic stroke in women: a prospective study. *JAMA.* 2000 Sep 27;284(12):1534–40.

13. Jacobs DR, Pereira MA, Meyer KA, Kushi LH. Fiber from whole grains, but not refined grains, is inversely associated with all-cause mortality in older women: the Iowa women's health study. *J Am Coll Nutr.* 2000 Jun;19(3 Suppl):326S–330S.

14. Bloch, A. et al. Position of the American Dietetic Association: Phytochemicals and functional foods. *JADA.* 1995;95:493–496.

15. McCullough ML, Robertson AS, Chao A, Jacobs EJ, Stampfer MJ, Jacobs DR, Diver WR, Calle EE, Thun MJ. A prospective study of whole grains, fruits, vegetables and colon cancer risk. *Cancer Causes Control.* 2003 Dec;14(10):959–70.

16. French L, Kendall S. Does a high-fiber diet prevent colon cancer in at-risk patients? *J Fam Pract.* 2003 Nov;52(11):892–3.

17. Hill M. Dietary fibre and colon cancer: where do we go from here? *Proc Nutr Soc.* 2003 Feb;62(1):63–5.

18. Carson JA. Nutrition therapy for dyslipidemia. *Curr Diab Rep.* 2003 Oct;3(5):397–403.

19. Anderson JW. Whole grains protect against atherosclerotic cardiovascular disease. *Proc Nutr Soc.* 2003 Feb;62(1):135–42.

20. Roma E, Adamidis D, Nikolara R, Constantopoulos A, Messaritakis J. Diet and chronic constipation in children: the role of fiber. *J Pediatr Gastroenterol Nutr.* 1999 Feb;28(2):169–74.

21. Lee AJ, Evans CJ, Hau CM, Fowkes FG. Fiber intake, constipation, and risk of varicose veins in the general population: Edinburgh Vein Study. *J Clin Epidemiol.* 2001 Apr;54(4):423–9.

22. Dapoigny M, Stockbrugger RW, Azpiroz F, Collins S, Coremans G, Muller-Lissner S, Oberndorff A, Pace F, Smout A, Vatn M, Whorwell P. Role of alimentation in irritable bowel syndrome. *Digestion.* 2003;67(4):225–33.

Chapter 6

1. National Academy of Sciences. 1982. Committee on Diet, Nutrition, and Cancer, assembly of Life Sciences, National Research Council, Diet, Nutrition and Cancer. Washington DC. National Academy Press.

2. Shahidi F, Naczk M. 1995. Food phenolics: sources, chemistry, effects, applications. Lancaster, PA: Technomic Publishing Company. Food phenolics: an overview; p 1–5.

3. Gonzalez-Paramas AM, Esteban-Ruano S, Santos-Buelga C, de Pascual-Teresa S, Rivas-Gonzalo JC. Flavanol content and antioxidant activity in winery byproducts. *J Agric Food Chem.* 2004 Jan 28;52(2):234–8.

4. Adom KK, Sorrells ME, Liu RH. Phytochemical profiles and antioxidant activity of wheat varieties. *J Agric Food Chem.* 2003 Dec 7;51(26):7825–34.

5. Burns J, Fraser PD, Bramley PM. Identification and quantification of carotenoids, tocopherols and chlorophylls in commonly consumed fruits and vegetables. *Phytochemistry.* 2003 Mar;62(6):939–47.

6. Kostyukovsky M, Rafaeli A, Gileadi C, Demchenko N, Shaaya E. Activation of octopaminergic receptors by essential oil

constituents isolated from aromatic plants: possible mode of action against insect pests. *Pest Manag Sci.* 2002 Nov;58(11):1101–6.

7. Huang Y, Chen SX, Ho SH. Bioactivities of methyl allyl disulfide and diallyl trisulfide from essential oil of garlic to two species of stored-product pests, Sitophilus zeamais (Coleoptera: Curculionidae) and Tribolium castaneum (Coleoptera: Tenebrionidae) *J Econ Entomol.* 2000 Apr;93(2):537–43.

8. Beckman KB, Ames BN. Endogenous oxidative damage of mtDNA. *Mutat Res.*1999 Mar 8;424(1-2):51–8.

9. Junqueira VB, Barros SB, Chan SS, Rodrigues L, Giavarotti L, Abud RL, Deucher GP. Aging and oxidative stress. *Mol Aspects Med.* 2004 Feb-Apr;25(1-2):5–16.

10. Kasapoglu M, Ozben T. Alterations of antioxidant enzymes and oxidative stress markers in aging. *Exp Gerontol.* 2001 Feb;36(2):209–20.

11. Rafael H. Cerebral atherosclerosis and oxidative stress in Alzheimer's disease. *J Alzheimers Dis.* 2003 Dec;5(6):479–80.

12. Serra JA, Marschoff ER, Dominguez RO, Guareschi EM, Famulari AL, Pagano MA, de Lustig ES; Collaborative Group for the Study of the Oxidative Stress, Argentina. Oxidative stress in Alzheimer's and vascular dementias: masking of the antioxidant profiles by a concomitant Type II diabetes mellitus condition. *J Neurol Sci.* 2004 Mar 15;218(1-2):17–24.

13. Aliev G, Smith MA, Obrenovich ME, de la Torre JC, Perry G. Role of vascular hypoperfusion-induced oxidative stress and mitochondria failure in the pathogenesis of Alzheimer's disease. *Neurotox Res.* 2003;5(7):491–504.

14. Flicker T, Green S. Comparison of Gas-Phase Free-Radical Populations in Tobacco Smoke and Model Systems by HPLC, *Environ Health Perspect.* 2001, 109:765–771.

15. O'Neill K, Murray B. Power plants, new evidence that nature's "phyto-fighters" are your best medicine. Woodland Publishing, 2002.

16. The Harvard Report on Cancer Prevention. Causes of human cancer. *Cancer Causes and Control.* 1996:7(1)S7–S9.

17. Doll R. Peto R. The Causes of Cancer. New York, NY: Oxford University Press, 1981.

18. National Vital Statistics Reports, Vol. 52, No. 9, November 7, 2003.

19. U.S. Census, 2003.

20. Steinmetz K, Potter J. Vegetables, fruit, and cancer prevention: a review. *J Am Diet Assoc.* 1996;96:1027–1039.

21. Block G, Patterson B, and Subar A. Fruit, vegetables, and cancer prevention: A review of epidemiological evidence. *Nutr and Cancer.* 1992; 18:1–29.

22. Liu RH. Protective role of phytochemicals in whole foods: implications for chronic disease prevention, *Applied Biotechnology, Food Science and Policy.* 2003;1(1)39–46.

23. Sun J, Chu Y-F, Wu X, Liu R. Antioxidant and antiproliferative activities of fruits. *J Agric Food Chem.* 2002 Dec 4;50(25):7449-54.

24. Eberhardt M, Lee C, Liu R. Antioxidant activity of fresh apples. *Nature.* 2000;405:903–904.

25. Jashipura K, Hu F, Monson J, et al. The effect of fruit and vegetable intake on risk for coronary heart disease. *Ann Int Med.* 2001;134:1106–1114.

26. Liu S, Lee IM, Ajani U, Cole SR, Buring JE, Manson JE; Physicians' Health Study. Intake of vegetables rich in carotenoids and risk of coronary heart disease in men: The Physicians' Health Study. *Int J Epidemiol.* 2001 Feb;30(1):130–5.

27. Liu S, Manson JE, Lee IM, Cole SR, Hennekens CH, Willett WC, Buring JE. Fruit and vegetable intake and risk of cardiovascular disease: the Women's Health Study. *Am J Clin Nutr.* 2000 Oct;72(4):922–8.

28. Joshipura KJ, Ascherio A, Manson JE, Stampfer MJ, Rimm EB, Speizer FE, Hennekens CH, Spiegelman D, Willett WC. Fruit and vegetable intake in relation to risk of ischemic stroke. *JAMA.* 1999 Oct 6;282(13):1233–9.

29. Conlin PR, Chow D, Miller ER 3rd, Svetkey LP, Lin PH, Harsha DW, Moore TJ, Sacks FM, Appel LJ. The effect of dietary patterns on blood pressure control in hypertensive patients: results from the Dietary Approaches to Stop Hypertension (DASH) trial. *Am J Hypertens.* 2000 Sep;13(9):949–55.

30. Steinberg D. Lewis A. Conner Memorial Lecture. Oxidative modification of LDL and atherogenesis. *Circulation.* 1997 Feb 18;95(4):1062–71.

31. Taylor A, Jacques PF, Epstein EM. Relations among aging, antioxidant status, and cataract. *Am J Clin Nutr.* 1995 Dec;62(6 Suppl):1439S–1447S.

32. Commenges D, Scotet V, Renaud S, Jacqmin-Gadda H, Barberger-Gateau P, Dartigues JF. Intake of flavonoids and risk of dementia. *Eur J Epidemiol.* 2000 Apr;16(4):357–63.

33. Riviere S, Lauque S, Vellas B. Health promotion programme: nutrition and Alzheimer's disease. *J Nutr Health Aging.* 1998;2(2):101–6.

34. La Rue A, Koehler KM, Wayne SJ, Chiulli SJ, Haaland KY, Garry PJ. Nutritional status and cognitive functioning in a normally aging sample: a 6-y reassessment. *Am J Clin Nutr.* 1997 Jan;65(1):20–9.

35. Smith W and others. Dietary oxidants and age-related maculopathy: The Blue Mountains Study. *Ophthalmology.* 1999;106:761–767.

36. Age-Related Eye Disease Study Research Group (AREDS). A randomized, placebo-controlled, clinical trial of high-dose supplementation with vitamins C and E, beta carotene, and zinc for age-related macular degeneration and

vision loss: AREDS report no. 8. *Archives of Ophthalmology*. 2001;119:1417–1436.

37. Ford ES, Mokdad AH. Fruit and vegetable consumption and diabetes mellitus incidence among U.S. adults. *Prev Med*. 2001 Jan;32(1):33–9.

38. Meyer KA, Kushi LH, Jacobs DR Jr, Slavin J, Sellers TA, Folsom AR. Carbohydrates, dietary fiber, and incident type 2 diabetes in older women. *Am J Clin Nutr*. 2000 Apr;71(4):921–30.

39. Epstein LH, Gordy CC, Raynor HA, Beddome M, Kilanowski CK, Paluch R. Increasing fruit and vegetable intake and decreasing fat and sugar intake in families at risk for childhood obesity. *Obes Res*. 2001 Mar;9(3):171–8.

40. Gartner C, Stahl W, Sies H. Lycopene is more bioavailable from tomato paste than from fresh tomatoes. *Am J Clin Nutr*. 1997;66:116–122.

41. Giovannucci E. Tomatoes, tomato-based products, lycopene, and cancer: review of the epidemiologic literature. *J Natl Cancer Inst*. 1999 Feb 17;91(4):317–31.

42. Position of the American Dietetic Association: phytochemicals and functional foods. *J Am Diet Assoc*. 1995 Apr;95(4):493–6.

43. Omenn GS, Goodman GE, Thornquist MD, Balmes J, Cullen MR, Glass A, Keogh JP, Meyskens FL, Valanis B, Williams JH, Barnhart S, Hammar S. Effects of a combination of beta carotene and vitamin A on lung cancer and cardiovascular disease. *N Engl J Med*. 1996 May 2;334(18):1150–5.

44. Podmore ID, Griffiths HR, Herbert K, Mistry N, Mistry P, Lunce J. Vitamin C exhibits pro-oxidant properties, *Nature*. 1998; 239:559.

45. Hennekens CH, Buring JE, Manson JE, Stampfer M, Rosner B, Cook NR, Belanger C, LaMotte F, Gaziano JM, Ridker PM, Willett W, Peto R. Lack of effect of long-term supplementation with beta carotene on the incidence of malignant neoplasms and cardiovascular disease. *N Engl J Med*. 1996 May 2;334(18):1145–9.

46. Blot WJ, Li JY, Taylor PR, Guo W, Dawsey S, Wang GQ, Yang CS, Zheng SF, Gail M, Li GY, et al. Nutrition intervention trials in Linxian, China: supplementation with specific vitamin/mineral combinations, cancer incidence, and disease-specific mortality in the general population. *J Natl Cancer Inst*. 1993 Sep 15;85(18):1483–92.

47. Stephens NG, Parsons A, Schofield PM, Kelly F, Cheeseman K, Mitchinson MJ. Randomised controlled trial of vitamin E in patients with coronary disease: Cambridge Heart Antioxidant Study (CHAOS) *Lancet*. 1996 Mar 23;347(9004):781–6.

48. Routine Vitamin supplementation to prevent cancer and cardiovascular disease. U.S. Preventive Services Task Force New Topic, 2003. http://www.ahrq.gov/clinic/3rduspstf/vitamins/vitaminsrr.htm

49. Fletcher RH, Fairfield KM. Vitamins for chronic disease prevention in adults: clinical applications. *JAMA*. 2002 Jun 19;287(23):3127–9.

Chapter 7

1. Broekmans WM, Klopping-Ketelaars IA, Weststrate JA, Tijburg LB, van Poppel G, Vink AA, Berendschot TT, Bots ML, Castenmiller WA, Kardinaal AF. Decreased carotenoid concentrations due to dietary sucrose polyesters do not affect possible markers of disease risk in humans. *J Nutr*. 2003 Mar;133(3):720-6.

2. Weststrate JA, van het Hof KH. Sucrose polyester and plasma carotenoid concentrations in healthy subjects. *Am J Clin Nutr*. 1995 Sep;62(3):591-7.

3. Welsch C. Relationship between dietary fat and experimental mammary tumorigenesis: a review and critique. *Cancer Res*. 1992; 52 (supplement):2040S-2048S.

4. Schaefer EJ. Lipoproteins, nutrition, and heart disease. *Am J Clin Nutr*. 2002 Feb;75(2):191-212.

5. Renaud S, Lanzmann-Petithory D. Coronary heart disease: dietary links and pathogenesis. *Public Health Nutr*. 2001 Apr;4(2B):459-74.

6. Nicolosi RJ, Wilson TA, Lawton C, Handelman GJ. Dietary effects on cardiovascular disease risk factors: beyond saturated fatty acids and cholesterol. *J Am Coll Nutr*. 2001 Oct;20(5 Suppl):421S-427S.

7. Prentice RL, Pepe M, Self SG. Dietary fat and breast cancer: a quantitative assessment of the epidemiological literature and a discussion of methodological issues. *Cancer Res*. 1989 Jun 15;49(12):3147-56.

8. Ornish D, Scherwitz LW, Billings JH, Brown SE, Gould KL, Merritt TA, Sparler S, Armstrong WT, Ports TA, Kirkeeide RL, Hogeboom C, Brand RJ. Intensive lifestyle changes for reversal of coronary heart disease. *JAMA*. 1998 Dec 16;280(23):2001–7.

9. Esselstyn CB Jr. Updating a 12-year experience with arrest and reversal therapy for coronary heart disease (an overdue requiem for palliative cardiology). *Am J Cardiol*. 1999 Aug 1;84(3):339–41.

10. Aldana SG, Greenlaw R, Diehl HA, Englert H, Jackson R.Impact of the coronary health improvement project (CHIP) on several employee populations. *J Occup Environ Med*. 2002 Sep;44(9):831–9.

11. Jequier E, Bray GA. Low-fat diets are preferred. *Am J Med*. 2002 Dec 30;113 Suppl 9B:41S-46S.

12. Continuing Survey of Food Intakes by Individuals, 1995, USDA.

13. Centers for Disease Control and Prevention (CDC). Trends in intake of energy and macronutrients—United States, 1971-2000. *MMWR Morb Mortal Wkly Rep*. 2004 Feb 6;53(4):80-2.

14. Behavioral Risk Factor Surveillance System, Centers for Disease Control, 2002. www.cdc. gov/brfss.

15. Nielsen SJ, Siega-Riz AM, Popkin BM. Trends in energy intake in U.S. between 1977 and 1996: similar shifts seen across age groups. *Obes Res* 2002;10:370-8.

16. Nielsen SJ, Popkin BM. Patterns and trends in food portion sizes, 1977–1998. *JAMA* 2003;289:450-3.

17. Hu FB, Stampfer MJ, Manson JE, Rimm E, Colditz GA, Rosner BA, Hennekens CH, Willett WC. Dietary fat intake and the risk of coronary heart disease in women. *N Engl J Med.* 1997 Nov 20;337(21):1491-9.

18. Jiang R, Manson JE, Stampfer MJ, Liu S, Willett WC, Hu FB. Nut and peanut butter consumption and risk of type 2 diabetes in women. *JAMA.* 2002 Nov 27;288(20):2554-60.

19. Harding AH, Day NE, Khaw KT, Bingham S, Luben R, Welsh A, Wareham NJ. Dietary fat and the risk of clinical type 2 diabetes: the European prospective investigation of Cancer-Norfolk study. *Am J Epidemiol.* 2004 Jan 1;159(1):73-82.

20. Hu FB, Willett WC. Optimal diets for prevention of coronary heart disease. *JAMA.* 2002 Nov 27;288(20):2569-78.

21. Dayton, S, Pearce M, Hashimoto S, Dixon W, Tomiyasu U. A controlled clinical trial of a diet high in unsaturated fat in preventing complications of atherosclerosis. *Circulation.* 1969;40(suppl 2);1-63.

22. Turpeinen O, Karvonen M, Pekkarinen M, Miettinen M, Elosuo R, Paavilainen E. Dietary prevention of coronary heart disease; the Finnish Mental Hospital Study. *Int J Empidemiol.* 1979;8:99-118.

23. Leren P. The Oslo Diet-Heart Study. *Acta Med Scand.* 1966;466(suppl):5-92.

24. Morris J, Ball K, Antonis A, et al. Controlled trial of soya-bean oil in myocardial infarction. *Lancet.* 1968;2:693-699.

25. Morris MC, Evans DA, Bienias JL, Tangney CC, Bennett DA, Wilson RS, Aggarwal N, Schneider J. Consumption of fish and n-3 fatty acids and risk of incident Alzheimer's disease. *Arch Neurol.* 2003 Jul;60(7):940-6.

26. Kushi L, Giovannucci E. Dietary fat and cancer. *Am J Med.* 2002 Dec 30;113 Suppl 9B:63S-70S.

27. de Lorgeril M, Salen P. Diet as preventive medicine in cardiology. *Curr Opin Cardiol.* 2000 Sep;15(5):364-70.

28. de Lorgeril M, Salen P, Martin JL, Monjaud I, Delaye J, Mamelle N. Mediterranean diet, traditional risk factors, and the rate of cardiovascular complications after myocardial infarction: final report of the Lyon Diet Heart Study. *Circulation.* 1999 Feb 16;99(6):779-85.

29. Jones PJ, Lau VW. Effect of n-3 polyunsaturated fatty acids on risk reduction of sudden death. *Nutr Rev.* 2002 Dec;60(12):407-9.

30. Lemaitre RN, King IB, Mozaffarian D, Kuller LH, Tracy RP, Siscovick DS. n-3 Polyunsaturated fatty acids, fatal ischemic heart disease, and nonfatal myocardial infarction in older adults: the Cardiovascular Health Study. *Am J Clin Nutr.* 2003 Feb;77(2):319-25.

31. Whelton SP, He J, Whelton PK, Muntner P. Meta-Analysis of observational studies on fish intake and coronary heart disease. *Am J Cardiol.* 2004 May 1;93(9):1119-23.

32. Marckmann P, Gronbaek M. Fish consumption and coronary heart disease mortality. A systematic review of prospective cohort studies. *Eur J Clin Nutr.* 1999 Aug;53(8):585-90.

33. Takahata K, Monobe K, Tada M, Weber PC. The benefits and risks of n-3 polyunsaturated fatty acids. *Biosci Biotechnol Biochem.* 1998 Nov;62(11):2079-85.

34. Lefevre M, Kris-Etherton PM, Zhao G, Tracy RP. Dietary fatty acids, hemostasis, and cardiovascular disease risk. *J Am Diet Assoc.* 2004 Mar;104(3):410-9.

35. Srinath Reddy K, Katan MB. Diet, nutrition and the prevention of hypertension and cardiovascular diseases. *Public Health Nutr.* 2004 Feb;7(1A):167-86.

36. Spence JD. Nutritional and metabolic aspects of stroke prevention. *Adv Neurol.* 2003;92:173-8.

37. Steyn NP, Mann J, Bennett PH, Temple N, Zimmet P, Tuomilehto J, Lindstrom J, Louheranta A. Diet, nutrition and the prevention of type 2 diabetes. *Public Health Nutr.* 2004 Feb;7(1A):147-65.

38. van Dam RM. The epidemiology of lifestyle and risk for type 2 diabetes. *Eur J Epidemiol.* 2003;18(12):1115-25.

39. Richter WO. Fatty acids and breast cancer—is there a relationship? *Eur J Med Res.* 2003 Aug 20;8(8):373-80.

40. Nkondjock A, Shatenstein B, Maisonneuve P, Ghadirian P. Specific fatty acids and human colorectal cancer: an overview. *Cancer Detect Prev.* 2003;27(1):55-66.

41. Lichtenstein AH, Kennedy E, Barrier P, Danford D, Ernst ND, Grundy SM, Leveille GA, Van Horn L, Williams CL, Booth SL. Dietary fat consumption and health. *Nutr Rev.* 1998 May;56(5 Pt 2):S3-19.

42. Cooper JL. Dietary lipids in the aetiology of Alzheimer's disease: implications for therapy. *Drugs Aging.* 2003;20(6):399-418.

43. Peet M. Nutrition and schizophrenia: an epidemiological and clinical perspective. *Nutr Health.* 2003;17(3):211-9.

44. Ascherio A, Rimm EB, Giovannucci EL, Spiegelman D, Stampfer M, Willett WC. Dietary fat and risk of coronary heart disease in men: cohort follow up study in the United States. *BMJ.* 1996 Jul 13;313(7049):84-90.

45. Pietinen P, Ascherio A, Korhonen P, Hartman AM, Willett WC, Albanes D,Virtamo J. Intake of

fatty acids and risk of coronary heart disease in a cohort of Finnish men. The Alpha-Tocopherol, Beta-Carotene Cancer Prevention Study. *Am J Epidemiol.* 1997 May 15;145(10):876-87.

46. Oomen CM, Ocke MC, Feskens EJ, van Erp-Baart MA, Kok FJ, Kromhout D. Association between trans fatty acid intake and 10-year risk of coronary heart disease in the Zutphen Elderly Study: a prospective population-based study. *Lancet.* 2001 Mar 10;357(9258):746-51.

47. Thom TJ, Epstein FH. Heart disease, cancer, and stroke mortality trends and their interrelations. An international perspective. *Circulation.* 1994 Jul;90(1):574-82.

48. Stender S, Dyerberg J. Influence of trans fatty acids on health. *Ann Nutr Metab.* 2004;48(2):61-6.

49. Salmeron J, Hu FB, Manson JE, Stampfer MJ, Colditz GA, Rimm EB, Willett WC. Dietary fat intake and risk of type 2 diabetes in women. *Am J Clin Nutr.* 2001 Jun;73(6):1019-26.

50. de Lorgeril M, Salen P. Dietary prevention of coronary heart disease: focus on omega-6/omega-3 essential fatty acid balance. *World Rev Nutr Diet.* 2003;92:57-73.

51. Alper CM, Mattes RD. Peanut consumption improves indices of cardiovascular disease risk in healthy adults. *J Am Coll Nutr.* 2003 Apr;22(2):133-41 .

52. Ros E, Nunez I, Perez-Heras A, Serra M, Gilabert R, Casals E, Deulofeu R. A walnut diet improves endothelial function in hypercholerolemic subjects: a randomized crossover trial. *Circulation.* 2004 Apr 6;109(13):1609-14.

53. Garg ML, Blake RJ, Wills RB. Macadamia nut consumption lowers plasma total and LDL cholesterol levels in hypercholesterolemic men. *J Nutr.* 2003 Apr;133(4):1060-3.

54. Jenkins DJ, Kendall CW, Marchie A, Faulkner DA, Wong JM, de Souza R, Emam A, Parker TL, Vidgen E, Lapsley KG, Trautwein EA, Josse RG, Leiter LA, Connelly PW. Effects of a dietary portfolio of cholesterol-lowering foods vs lovastatin on serum lipids and C-reactive protein. *JAMA.* 2003 Jul 23;290(4):502-10.

55. Sicherer SH, Munoz-Furlong A, Sampson HA. Prevalence of peanut and tree nut allergy in the United States determined by means of a random digit dial telephone survey: a 5-year follow-up study. *J Allergy Clin Immunol.* 2003 Dec;112(6):1203-7.

56. Garcia-Lorda P, Megias Rangil I, Salas-Salvado J. Nut consumption, body weight and insulin resistance. *Eur J Clin Nutr.* 2003 Sep;57 Suppl 1: S8-11.

57. Sabate J. Nut consumption and body weight. *Am J Clin Nutr.* 2003 Sep;78(3 Suppl):647S-650S.

58. FDA Consumer magazine, Revealing Trans Fats. September-October 2003 Issue, Pub No. FDA03-1329C on the Web at http://www.fda.gov/fdac/features/2003/503_fats.html

59. Ballew C, Kuester S, Gillespie C. Beverage choices affect adequacy of children's nutrient intakes. *Arch Pediatr Adolesc Med.* 2000 Nov;154(11):1148-52.

60. French SA, Story M, Fulkerson JA, Gerlach AF. Food environment in secondary schools: a la carte, vending machines, and food policies and practices. *Am J Public Health.* 2003 Jul;93(7):1161-7.

61. Sanders TH. Non-detectable levels of trans-fatty acids in peanut butter. *J Agric Food Chem.* 2001 May;49(5):2349-51.

62. Allison DB, Egan SK, Barraj LM, Caughman C, Infante M, Heimbach JT. Estimated intakes of trans fatty and other fatty acids in the US population. *J Am Diet Assoc.* 1999 Feb;99(2):166-74.

63. Willett W. Eat Drink and Be Healthy: the Harvard Medical School guide to healthy eating. 2001, Simon and Schuster Source, New York, NY.

64. Kochanek KD, Smith BL. Deaths: preliminary data for 2002. *Natl Vital Stat Rep.* 2004 Feb 11;52(13):1-47.

Chapter 8

1. van Dam RM, Rimm EB, Willett WC, Stampfer MJ, Hu FB. Dietary patterns and risk for type 2 diabetes mellitus in U.S. men. *Ann Intern Med.* 2002 Feb 5;136(3):201–9.

2. Hu FB, Manson JE, Stampfer MJ, Colditz G, Liu S, Solomon CG, Willett WC. Diet, lifestyle, and the risk of type 2 diabetes mellitus in women. *N Engl J Med.* 2001 Sep 13;345(11):790–7.

3. Fung TT, Willett WC, Stampfer MJ, Manson JE, Hu FB. Dietary patterns and the risk of coronary heart disease in women. *Arch Intern Med.* 2001 Aug 13-27;161(15):1857–62.

4. Hu FB, Rimm EB, Stampfer MJ, Ascherio A, Spiegelman D, Willett WC. Prospective study of major dietary patterns and risk of coronary heart disease in men. *Am J Clin Nutr.* 2000 Oct;72(4):912–21.

5. Schulze MB, Hu FB. Dietary patterns and risk of hypertension, type 2 diabetes mellitus, and coronary heart disease. *Curr Atheroscler Rep.* 2002 Nov;4(6):462–7.

6. Millen BE, Quatromoni PA, Nam BH, O'Horo CE, Polak JF, Wolf PA, D'Agostino RB; Framingham Nutrition Studies. Dietary patterns, smoking, and subclinical heart disease in women: opportunities for primary prevention from the Framingham Nutrition Studies. *J Am Diet Assoc.* 2004 Feb;104(2):208–14.

7. Fung TT, Rimm EB, Spiegelman D, Rifai N, Tofler GH, Willett WC, Hu FB. Association between dietary patterns and plasma biomarkers of obesity and cardiovascular disease risk. *Am J Clin Nutr.* 2001 Jan;73(1):61–7.

8. Terry P, Hu FB, Hansen H, Wolk A. Prospective study of major dietary patterns and colorectal

cancer risk in women. *Am J Epidemiol.* 2001 Dec 15;154(12):1143–9.

9. Terry P, Suzuki R, Hu FB, Wolk A. A prospective study of major dietary patterns and the risk of breast cancer. *Cancer Epidemiol Biomarkers Prev.* 2001 Dec;10(12):1281–5.

10. Norat T, Riboli E. Meat consumption and colorectal cancer: a review of epidemiologic evidence. *Nutr Rev.* 2001 Feb;59(2):37–47.

11. Truswell AS. Meat consumption and cancer of the large bowel. *Eur J Clin Nutr.* 2002 Mar;56 Suppl 1:S19–24.

12. Hill M. Meat, cancer and dietary advice to the public. *Eur J Clin Nutr.* 2002 Mar;56 Suppl 1: S36–4.

13. Missmer SA, Smith-Warner SA, Spiegelman D, Yaun SS, Adami HO, Beeson WL, van den Brandt PA, Fraser GE, Freudenheim JL, Goldbohm RA, Graham S, Kushi LH, Miller AB, Potter JD, Rohan TE, Speizer FE, Toniolo P, Willett WC, Wolk A, Zeleniuch-Jacquotte A, Hunter DJ. Meat and dairy food consumption and breast cancer: a pooled analysis of cohort studies. *Int J Epidemiol.* 2002 Feb;31(1):78–85.

14. Cho E, Spiegelman D, Hunter DJ, Chen WY, Stampfer MJ, Colditz GA, Willett WC. Premenopausal fat intake and risk of breast cancer. *J Natl Cancer Inst.* 2003 Jul 16;95(14):1079–85.

15. Fraser GE, Shavlik DJ. Ten years of life: Is it a matter of choice? *Arch Intern Med.* 2001 Jul 9;161(13):1645–52.

16. Singh PN, Sabate J, Fraser GE. Does low meat consumption increase life expectancy in humans? *Am J Clin Nutr.* 2003 Sep;78(3 Suppl):526S–532S.

17. Fraser GE. Determinants of ischemic heart disease in Seventh-day Adventists: a review. *Am J Clin Nutr.* 1988 Sep;48(3 Suppl):833–6.

18. Ascherio A. Willett W, Rimm E, Giovannucci E, Stampfer M. Dietary iron intake and risk of coronary disease among men. *Circulation,* 1994;89:969–74.

19. Key TJ, Schatzkin A, Willett WC, Allen NE, Spencer EA, Travis RC. Diet, nutrition and the prevention of cancer. *Public Health Nutr.* 2004 Feb;7(1A):187–200.

20. Sugimura T. Food and cancer. *Toxicology.* 2002 Dec 27;181–182:17–21.

21. Mitra AK, Faruque FS, Avis AL. Breast cancer and environmental risks: where is the link? *Environ Health.* 2004 Mar;66(7):24–32,40.

22. Willett WC, Sacks F, Trichopoulou A, Drescher G, Ferro-Luzzi A, Helsing E, Trichopoulos D. Mediterranean diet pyramid: a cultural model for healthy eating. *Am J Clin Nutr.* 1995 Jun;61(6 Suppl):1402S–1406S.

23. Weggemans RM, Zock PL, Katan MB. Dietary cholesterol from eggs increases the ratio of total cholesterol to high-density lipoprotein cholesterol in humans: a meta-analysis. *Am J*

Clin Nutr. 2001 May;73(5):885–91.

24. Kritchevsky SB, Kritchevsky D. Egg consumption and coronary heart disease: an epidemiologic overview. *J Am Coll Nutr.* 2000 Oct;19(5 Suppl):549S–555S.

25. McNamara DJ. The impact of egg limitations on coronary heart disease risk: do the numbers add up? *J Am Coll Nutr.* 2000 Oct;19(5 Suppl):540S–548S.

26. Weinsier RL, Krumdieck CL. Dairy foods and bone health: examination of the evidence. *Am J Clin Nutr.* 2000 Sep;72(3):681–9.

27. Millen BE, Quatromoni PA, Nam BH, O'Horo CE, Polak JF, Wolf PA, D'Agostino RB; Framingham Nutrition Studies. Dietary patterns, smoking, and subclinical heart disease in women: opportunities for primary prevention from the Framingham Nutrition Studies. *J Am Diet Assoc.* 2004 Feb;104(2):208–14.

28. Norat T, Riboli E. Dairy products and colorectal cancer. A review of possible mechanisms and epidemiological evidence. *Eur J Clin Nutr.* 2003 Jan;57(1):1–17.

29. Shin MH, Holmes MD, Hankinson SE, Wu K, Colditz GA, Willett WC. Intake of dairy products, calcium, and vitamin D and risk of breast cancer. *J Natl Cancer Inst.* 2002 Sep 4;94(17):1301–11.

30. Chan JM, Giovannucci EL. Dairy products, calcium, and vitamin D and risk of prostate cancer. *Epidemiol Rev.* 2001;23(1):87-92.

31. Dagnelie PC, Schuurman AG, Goldbohm RA, Van Den Brandt PA.Diet, anthropometric measures and prostate cancer risk: a review of prospective cohort and intervention studies. *BJU Int.* 2004 May;93(8):1139–50.

32. Ghadirian P, Lynch HT, Krewski D. Epidemiology of pancreatic cancer: an overview. *Cancer Detect Prev.* 2003;27(2):87–93.

33. Host A. Frequency of cow's milk allergy in childhood. *Ann Allergy Asthma Immunol.* 2002 Dec;89(6 Suppl 1):33–7.

34. Menotti A, Kromhout D, Blackburn H, Fidanza F, Buzina R, Nissinen A. Food intake patterns and 25-year mortality from coronary heart disease: cross-cultural correlations in the Seven Countries Study. The Seven Countries Study Research Group. *Eur J Epidemiol.* 1999 Jul;15(6):507–15.

35. Hu FB, Stampfer MJ, Manson JE, Rimm E, Colditz GA, Speizer FE, Hennekens CH, Willett WC. Dietary protein and risk of ischemic heart disease in women. *Am J Clin Nutr.* 1999 Aug;70(2):221-7.

36. Elwood PC, Pickering JE, Hughes J, Fehily AM, Ness AR. Milk drinking, ischaemic heart disease and ischaemic stroke II. Evidence from cohort studies. *Eur J Clin Nutr.* 2004 May;58(5):718–24.

37. Obarzanek E, Sacks FM, Vollmer WM, Bray GA, Miller ER 3rd, Lin PH, Karanja NM, Most-

Windhauser MM, Moore TJ, Swain JF, Bales CW, Proschan MA; DASH Research Group. Effects on blood lipids of a blood pressure-lowering diet: the Dietary Approaches to Stop Hypertension (DASH) Trial. *Am J Clin Nutr.* 2001 Jul;74(1):80–9.

38. Pi-Sunyer FX. Glycemic index and disease. *Am J Clin Nutr.* 2002 Jul;76(1):290S–8S

39. Rizkalla SW, Bellisle F, Slama G. Health benefits of low glycaemic index foods, such as pulses, in diabetic patients and healthy individuals. *Br J Nutr.* 2002 Dec;88 Suppl 3: S255–62.

40. Brand-Miller JC, Holt SH, Pawlak DB, McMillan J. Glycemic index and obesity. *Am J Clin Nutr.* 2002 Jul;76(1):281S–5S.

41. Roberts SB. Glycemic index and satiety. *Nutr Clin Care.* 2003 Jan-Apr;6(1):20–6.

42. Willett W, Manson J, Liu S. Glycemic index, glycemic load, and risk of type 2 diabetes. *Am J Clin Nutr.* 2002 Jul;76(1):274S–80S.

43. Leeds AR. Glycemic index and heart disease. *Am J Clin Nutr.* 2002 Jul;76(1):286S–9S.

44. Jenkins DJ, Kendall CW, Augustin LS, Franceschi S, Hamidi M, Marchie A, Jenkins AL, Axelsen M. Glycemic index: overview of implications in health and disease. *Am J Clin Nutr.* 2002 Jul;76(1):266S–73S.

45. Reynolds K, Lewis B, Nolen JD, Kinney GL, Sathya B, He J. Alcohol consumption and risk of stroke: a meta-analysis. *JAMA.* 2003 Feb 5;289(5):579–88.

46. Corrao G, Bagnardi V, Zambon A, La Vecchia C. A meta-analysis of alcohol consumption and the risk of 15 diseases. *Prev Med.* 2004 May;38(5):613–9.

47. Corrao G, Rubbiati L, Bagnardi V, Zambon A, Poikolainen K. Alcohol and coronary heart disease: a meta-analysis. *Addiction.* 2000 Oct;95(10):1505–23.

48. Bagnardi V, Blangiardo M, La Vecchia C, Corrao G. A meta-analysis of alcohol drinking and cancer risk. *Br J Cancer.* 2001 Nov 30;85(11):1700–5.

49. Anderson P, Cremona A, Paton A, Turner C, Wallace P. The risk of alcohol. *Addiction.* 1993 Nov;88(11):1493–508.

50. Bagnardi V, Blangiardo M, La Vecchia C, Corrao G. Alcohol consumption and the risk of cancer: a meta-analysis. *Alcohol Res Health.* 2001;25(4):263–70.

Chapter 9

1. Behavioral Risk Factor Surveillance System, Centers for Disease Control, 2000. www.cdc.gov/brfss.

2. Behavioral Risk Factor Surveillance System, Centers for Disease Control, 1990–2002. www.cdc.gov/brfss.

3. Blair SN, Cheng Y, Holder JS. Is physical activity or physical fitness more important in defining health benefits? *Med Sci Sports Exerc.* 2001 Jun;33(6 Suppl):S379–99.

4. Williams PT. Physical fitness and activity as separate heart disease risk factors: a meta-analysis. *Med Sci Sports Exerc.* 2001 May;33(5):754–61.

5. Berlin JA, Colditz GA. A meta-analysis of physical activity in the prevention of coronary heart disease. *Am J Epidemiol.* 1990 Oct;132(4):612–28.

6. Batty GD. Physical activity and coronary heart disease in older adults. A systematic review of epidemiological studies. *Eur J Public Health.* 2002 Sep;12(3):171–6.

7. Blair SN, Kohl HW 3rd, Paffenbarger RS Jr, Clark DG, Cooper KH, Gibbons LW. Physical fitness and all-cause mortality. A prospective study of healthy men and women. *JAMA.* 1989 Nov 3;262(17):2395–401.

8. Katzmarzyk PT, Janssen I, Ardern CI. Physical inactivity, excess adiposity and premature mortality. *Obes Rev.* 2003 Nov;4(4):257–90.

9. Myers J, Prakash M, Froelicher V, Do D, Partington S, Atwood JE. Exercise capacity and mortality among men referred for exercise testing. *N Engl J Med.* 2002 Mar 14;346(11):793-801.

10. Lee CD, Folsom AR, Blair SN. Physical activity and stroke risk: a meta-analysis. *Stroke.* 2003 Oct;34(10):2475–81.

11. Moyna NM, Thompson PD. The effect of physical activity on endothelial function in man. *Acta Physiol Scand.* 2004 Feb;180(2):113–23.

12. Durstine JL, Grandjean PW, Davis PG, Ferguson MA, Alderson NL, DuBose KD. Blood lipid and lipoprotein adaptations to exercise: a quantitative analysis. *Sports Med.* 2001;31(15):1033–62.

13. Szapary PO, Bloedon LT, Foster GD. Physical activity and its effects on lipids. *Curr Cardiol Rep.* 2003 Nov;5(6):488–92.

14. Chobanian AV, et al. Seventh report of the Joint National Committee on Prevention, Detection, Evaluation, and Treatment of High Blood Pressure. *Hypertension.* 2003 Dec;42(6):1206–52.

15. Whelton SP, Chin A, Xin X, He J. Effect of aerobic exercise on blood pressure: a meta-analysis of randomized, controlled trials. *Ann Intern Med.* 2002 Apr 2;136(7):493–503.

16. Lesniak KT, Dubbert PM. Exercise and hypertension. *Curr Opin Cardiol.* 2001 Nov;16(6):356–9.

17. Peirce NS. Diabetes and exercise. *Br J Sports Med.* 1999 Jun;33(3):161–72.

18. Kelley DE, Goodpaster BH. Effects of physical activity on insulin action and glucose tolerance in obesity. *Med Sci Sports Exerc.* 1999 Nov;31(11 Suppl):S619–23.

19. Robinson DM, Ogilvie RW, Tullson PC, Terjung RL. Increased peak oxygen consumption of

trained muscle requires increased electron flux capacity. *J Appl Physiol.* 1994 Oct;77(4):1941–52.

20. Rennie MJ, Wackerhage H, Spangenburg EE, Booth FW. Control of the size of the human muscle mass. *Annu Rev Physiol.* 2004;66:799–828.

21. Lee IM. Physical activity and cancer prevention—data from epidemiologic studies. *Med Sci Sports Exerc.* 2003 Nov;35(11):1823–7.

22. Westerlind KC. Physical activity and cancer prevention–mechanisms. *Med Sci Sports Exerc.* 2003 Nov;35(11):1834–40.

23. Quadrilatero J, Hoffman-Goetz L. Physical activity and colon cancer: a systematic review of potential mechanisms. *J Sports Med Phys Fitness.* 2003 Jun;43(2):121–38.

24. Friedenreich CM. Physical activity and cancer prevention: from observational to intervention research. *Cancer Epidemiol Biomarkers Prev.* 2001 Apr;10(4):287–301.

25. McTiernan A. Physical activity after cancer: physiologic outcomes. *Cancer Invest.* 2004;22(1):68–81.

26. Boyde A. The real response of bone to exercise *J Anat.* 2003 Aug;203(2):173–89.

27. Beck BR, Snow CM. Bone health across the lifespan—exercising our options. *Exerc Sport Sci Rev.* 2003 Jul;31(3):117–22.

28. Kessenich C. An approach to postmenopausal osteoporosis treatment: a case study review. *J Am Acad Nurse Pract.* 2003 Dec;15(12):539–45.

29. Droppert PM. The effects of microgravity on the skeletal system—a review. *J Br Interplanet Soc.* 1990 Jan;43(1):19–24.

30. Paluska SA, Schwenk TL. Physical activity and mental health: current concepts. *Sports Med.* 2000 Mar;29(3):167–80.

31. Goodwin RD. Association between physical activity and mental disorders among adults in the United States. *Prev Med.* 2003 Jun;36(6):698–703.

32. Dunn AL, Trivedi MH, O'Neal HA. Physical activity dose-response effects on outcomes of depression and anxiety. *Med Sci Sports Exerc.* 2001 Jun;33(6 Suppl):S587–97.

33. Fox KR. The influence of physical activity on mental well-being. *Public Health Nutr.* 1999 Sep;2(3A):411–8.

34. Crews DJ, Landers DM. A meta-analytic review of aerobic fitness and reactivity to psychosocial stressors. *Med Sci Sports Exerc.* 1987 Oct;19(5 Suppl):S114–20.

35. Sherrill DL, Kotchou K, Quan SF. Association of physical activity and human sleep disorders. *Arch Intern Med.* 1998 Sep 28;158(17):1894–8.

36. O'Connor PJ, Youngstedt SD. Influence of exercise on human sleep. *Exerc Sport Sci Rev.* 1995;23:105–34.

37. Larsen GE, George JD, Alexander JL, Fellingham GW, Aldana SG, Parcell AC. Prediction of maximum oxygen consumption from walking, jogging, or running. *Res Q Exerc Sport.* 2002 Mar;73(1):66–72.

Chapter 10

1. King KM, Humen DP, Teo KK. Cardiac rehabilitation: the forgotten intervention. *Can J Cardiol.* 1999 Sep;15(9):979–85.

2. American College of Sports Medicine position stand. The recommended quantity and quality of exercise for developing and maintaining cardiorespiratory and muscular fitness in healthy adults. *Med Sci Sports Exerc.* 1990 Apr;22(2):265–74.

3. DeBusk RF, Stenestrand U, Sheehan M, Haskell WL. Training effects of long versus short bouts of exercise in healthy subjects. *Am J Cardiol.* 1990 Apr 15;65(15):1010–3.

4. Ebisu T. Splitting the distance of endurance running on cardiovascular endurance and blood lipids. *Japanese Journal of Physical Education.* 1985 30:37–43.

5. Pate RR, Pratt M, Blair SN, Haskell WL, Macera CA, Bouchard C, Buchner D, Ettinger W, Heath GW, King AC, et al. Physical activity and public health. A recommendation from the Centers for Disease Control and Prevention and the American College of Sports Medicine. *JAMA.* 1995 Feb 1;273(5):402–7.

6. Tanaka H, Monahan KD, Seals DR. Age-predicted maximal heart rate revisited. *J Am Coll Cardiol.* 2001 Jan;37(1):153–6.

7. Eskurza I, Donato AJ, Moreau KL, Seals DR, Tanaka H. Changes in maximal aerobic capacity with age in endurance-trained women: 7-yr follow-up. *J Appl Physiol.* 2002 Jun;92(6):2303–8.

8. Hawkins S, Wiswell R. Rate and mechanism of maximal oxygen consumption decline with aging: implications for exercise training. *Sports Med.* 2003;33(12):877–88.

9. McGuire DK, Levine BD, Williamson JW, Snell PG, Blomqvist CG, Saltin B, Mitchell JH. A 30-year follow-up of the Dallas Bedrest and Training Study: I. Effect of age on the cardiovascular response to exercise. *Circulation.* 2001 Sep 18;104(12):1350–7.

10. McGuire DK, Levine BD, Williamson JW, Snell PG, Blomqvist CG, Saltin B, Mitchell JH. A 30-year follow-up of the Dallas Bedrest and Training Study: II. Effect of age on cardiovascular adaptation to exercise training. *Circulation.* 2001 Sep 18;104(12):1358–66.

11. Kujala UM, Kaprio J, Sarna S, Koskenvuo M. Relationship of leisure-time physical activity and mortality: the Finnish twin cohort. *JAMA.* 1998 Feb 11;279(6):440–4.

12. Maes HH, Beunen GP, Vlietinck RF, Neale MC, Thomis M, Vanden Eynde B, Lysens R, Simons J, Derom C, Derom R. Inheritance of physical fitness in 10-yr-old twins and their parents. *Med Sci Sports Exerc.* 1996 Dec;28(12):1479–91.

13. Heymsfield SB, Gallagher D, Visser M, Nunez C, Wang ZM. Measurement of skeletal muscle: laboratory and epidemiological methods. *J Gerontol A Biol Sci Med Sci.* 1995 Nov;50 Spec No:23–9.

14. Tarpenning KM, Hamilton-Wessler M, Wiswell RA, Hawkins SA. Endurance training delays age of decline in leg strength and muscle morphology. *Med Sci Sports Exerc.* 2004 Jan;36(1):74–8.

15. Macaluso A, De Vito G. Muscle strength, power and adaptations to resistance training in older people. *Eur J Appl Physiol.* 2004 Apr;91(4):450–72.

16. Latham NK, Bennett DA, Stretton CM, Anderson CS. Systematic review of progressive resistance strength training in older adults. *J Gerontol A Biol Sci Med Sci.* 2004 Jan;59(1):48–61.

17. Centers for Disease Control and Prevention (CDC). Strength training among adults aged over 65 years—United States, 2001. *MMWR Morb Mortal Wkly Rep.* 2004 Jan 23;53(2):25–8.

18. Hass CJ, Feigenbaum MS, Franklin BA. Prescription of resistance training for healthy populations. *Sports Med.* 2001;31(14):953–64.

Chapter 11

1. DiClemente CC, Prochaska JO, Fairhurst SK, Velicer WF, Velasquez MM, Rossi JS. The process of smoking cessation: an analysis of precontemplation, contemplation, and preparation stages of change. *J Consult Clin Psychol.* 1991 Apr;59(2):295–304.

2. Prochaska JO, DiClemente CC. Stages and processes of self-change of smoking: toward an integrative model of change. *J Consult Clin Psychol.* 1983 Jun;51(3):390–5.

3. Bandura A. Social foundations of thought and action: a social cognitive theory. 1986, Englewood Cliffs, NJ: Prentice Hall.

4. Sarason I, Sarason B. Social support: Theory, research, and applications. 1985, The Hague: Martinus Nijhoff.

5. Janis I, Mann L. Decision making: a psychological analysis of conflict, choice, and commitment. 1977, New York: Collier Macmillan.

6. Simpson ME, Serdula M, Galuska DA, Gillespie C, Donehoo R, Macera C, Mack K. Walking trends among U.S. adults: the Behavioral Risk Factor Surveillance System, 1987-2000. *Am J Prev Med.* 2003 Aug;25(2):95–100.

7. Eyler AA, Brownson RC, Bacak SJ, Housemann RA. The epidemiology of walking for physical activity in the United States. *Med Sci Sports Exerc.* 2003 Sep;35(9):1529–36.

8. Bandura A. Health promotion by social cognitive means. *Health Educ Behav.* 2004 Apr;31(2):143–64.

9. McAuley E, Blissmer B. Self-efficacy determinants and consequences of physical activity. *Exerc Sport Sci Rev.* 2000 Apr;28(2):85–8.

10. Marcus B, Forsyth L. Motivating people to be physically active. 2003, Human Kinetics, Champaign, IL.

11. Hoelscher D, Day R, Lee E, Frankowski R, Kelder S, Ward J, Scheurer M. Measuring the Prevalence of Overweight in Texas Schoolchildren. *Am J Public Health* 2004 94: 1002–1008.

Chapter 12

1. Glanz K, Basil M, Maibach E, Goldberg J, Snyder D. Why Americans eat what they do: taste, nutrition, cost, convenience, and weight control concerns as influences on food consumption. *J Am Diet Assoc.* 1998 Oct;98(10):1118–26.

2. Ma J, Betts NM, Horacek T, Georgiou C, White A, Nitzke S. The importance of decisional balance and self-efficacy in relation to stages of change for fruit and vegetable intakes by young adults. *Am J Health Promot.* 2002 Jan–Feb;16(3):157–66.

3. Kumanyika SK, Van Horn L, Bowen D, Perri MG, Rolls BJ, Czajkowski SM, Schron E. Maintenance of dietary behavior change. *Health Psychol.* 2000 Jan;19(1 Suppl):42–56.

4. Campbell MK, Reynolds KD, Havas S, Curry S, Bishop D, Nicklas T, Palombo R, Buller D, Feldman R, Topor M, Johnson C, Beresford SA, Motsinger BM, Morrill C, Heimendinger J. Stages of change for increasing fruit and vegetable consumption among adults and young adults participating in the National 5-a-Day for Better Health community studies. *Health Educ Behav.* 1999 Aug;26(4):513–34.

5. Shepherd R, Shepherd R. Resistance to changes in diet. *Proc Nutr Soc.* 2002 May;61(2):267–72.

6. Ling A, Horwath C. Perceived benefits and barriers of increased fruit and vegetable consumption: validation of a decisional balance scale. *J Nutr Educ.* 2001 Sep–Oct;33(5):257–65.

7. Slavin JL, Jacobs D, Marquart L, Wiemer K. The role of whole grains in disease prevention. *J Am Diet Assoc.* 2001 Jul;101(7):780–5.

8. Lin B, Guthrie J, Frazao E. Nutrient contribution of food away from home. In: America's Eating Habits: Changes and Consequences, 1999, pages 213–242. U.S. Department of Agriculture, Economic Research Service, Washington, D.C. Agriculture Information Bulletin No. 750.

9. French SA, Story M, Jeffery RW. Environmental influences on eating and physical activity. *Annu Rev Public Health.* 2001;22:309–35.

10. Frazao ZE. America's eating habits: changes and consequences. 1999, Washington, D.C.: USDA/Econ. Res. Serv.

11. Jacobson M. *Liquid Candy: How soft drinks are harming American's healthy.* Washington, D.C.: Center for Science in the Public Interest, 1998.

12. Kraak V, Pelletier D. The influence of commercialism on the food purchasing behavior of children and teenage youth. *Fam Econ Nutr Rev.* 1998;11:15–24.

13. Advertising Age. Leading National Advertisers, 1999, on the Web at: www.adage.com

14. Jeffery R, French S, Schmid T. Attributions for dietary failures: problems reported by participants in the hypertension prevention trial. *Health Psychol.* 1990;9:315–329.

15. Brownell K, Rodin J. The weight maintenance survival guide. Dallas: American Health Publishing; 1990.

16. Brownell KD, Cohen LR. Adherence to dietary regimens. 2: Components of effective interventions. *Behav Med.* 1995 Winter;20(4):155–64.

17. Cullen KW, Baranowski T, Smith SP. Using goal setting as a strategy for dietary behavior change. *J Am Diet Assoc.* 2001 May;101(5):562–6.

Chapter 13

1. CDC, National Center for Health Statistics, National Health and Nutrition Examination Survey. Health, United States (Table 70) 2002.

2. Kruger J, Galuska DA, Serdula MK, Jones DA. Attempting to lose weight: specific practices among U.S. adults. *Am J Prev Med.* 2004 Jun;26(5):402–6.

3. Serdula MK, Mokdad AH, Williamson DF, Galuska DA, Mendlein JM, Heath GW. Prevalence of attempting weight loss and strategies for controlling weight. *JAMA.* 1999 Oct 13;282(14):1353–8.

4. Appel LJ, Champagne CM, Harsha DW, Cooper LS, Obarzanek E, Elmer PJ, Stevens VJ, Vollmer WM, Lin PH, Svetkey LP, Stedman SW, Young DR; Writing Group of the PREMIER Collaborative Research Group. Effects of comprehensive lifestyle modification on blood pressure control: main results of the PREMIER clinical trial. *JAMA.* 2003 Apr 23–30;289(16):2083–93.

5. Esposito K, Giugliano F, Di Palo C, Giugliano G, Marfella R, D'Andrea F, D'Armiento M, Giugliano D. Effect of lifestyle changes on erectile dysfunction in obese men: a randomized controlled trial. *JAMA.* 2004 Jun 23;291(24):2978–84.

6. Knowler WC, Barrett-Connor E, Fowler SE, Hamman RF, Lachin JM, Walker EA, Nathan DM; Diabetes Prevention Program Research Group. Reduction in the incidence of type 2 diabetes with lifestyle intervention or metformin. *N Engl J Med.* 2002 Feb 7;346(6):393–403.

7. Kumanyika SK, Van Horn L, Bowen D, Perri MG, Rolls BJ, Czajkowski SM, Schron E. Maintenance of dietary behavior change. *Health Psychol.* 2000 Jan;19(1 Suppl):42–56.

8. French SA, Story M, Jeffery RW. Environmental influences on eating and physical activity. *Annu Rev Public Health* 2001;22:309–35.

9. Wadden TA, Brownell KD, Foster GD. Obesity: responding to the global epidemic. *J Consult Clin Psychol* 2002 Jun;70(3):510–25.

10. Wright J, Kennedy-Stephenson J, Wang C, McDowell M, Johnson C, Trends in Intake of Energy and Macronutrients—United States, 1971—2000, *MMWR,* February 6, 2004 / 53(04);80–82. On the Web at: http://www.cdc.gov/mmwr/preview/mmwrhtml/mm5304a3.htm

11. Putnam J. Major trends in the U.S. food supply. *Food Rev.* 2000 23–13.

12. Frazao ZE. America's eating habits: changes and consequences. 1999, Washington, D.C.: USDA/Econ. Res. Serv. 71–95.

13. Young LR, Nestle M. The contribution of expanding portion sizes to the U.S. obesity epidemic. *Am J Public Health.* 2002 Feb;92(2):246–9.

14. Wansink B. Can package size accelerate usage volume? *J Marketing.* 1996 60:1–13.

15. Rolls B, Engell D, Birch L. Serving portion size influences 5-year-old but not 3-year-old children's food intakes. *J Am Diet Assoc.* 2000 100:232–234.

16. Guthrie JF, Morton JF. Food sources of added sweeteners in the diets of Americans. *J Am Diet Assoc.* 2000 Jan;100(1):43–51.

17. Kramer FM, Jeffery RW, Forster JL, Snell MK. Long-term follow-up of behavioral treatment for obesity: patterns of weight regain among men and women. *Int J Obes.* 1989;13(2):123–36.

18. Weinsier RL, Nagy TR, Hunter GR, Darnell BE, Hensrud DD, Weiss HL. Do adaptive changes in metabolic rate favor weight regain in weight-reduced individuals? An examination of the set-point theory. *Am J Clin Nutr.* 2000 Nov;72(5):1088–94.

19. Ross R, Janssen I, Tremblay A. Obesity reduction through lifestyle modification. *Can J Appl Physiol.* 2000 Feb;25(1):1–18.

20. Klem ML, Wing RR, McGuire MT, Seagle HM, Hill JO. A descriptive study of individuals successful at long-term maintenance of substantial weight loss. *Am J Clin Nutr.* 1997 Aug;66(2):239–46.

21. Phelan S, Hill JO, Lang W, Dibello JR, Wing RR. Recovery from relapse among successful weight maintainers. *Am J Clin Nutr.* 2003 Dec;78(6):1079–84.

22. Wyatt HR, Grunwald GK, Mosca CL, Klem ML, Wing RR, Hill JO. Long-term weight loss and breakfast in subjects in the National Weight Control Registry. *Obes Res.* 2002 Feb;10(2):78–82.

23. Wing RR, Hill JO. Successful weight loss maintenance. *Annu Rev Nutr.* 2001;21:323–41.

24. Shick SM, Wing RR, Klem ML, McGuire MT, Hill JO, Seagle H. Persons successful at long-term weight loss and maintenance continue to consume a low-energy, low-fat diet. *J Am Diet Assoc.* 1998 Apr;98(4):408–13.

25. McGuire MT, Wing RR, Klem ML, Hill JO. Behavioral strategies of individuals who have maintained long-term weight losses. *Obes Res.* 1999 Jul;7(4):334–41.

26. The truth about dieting. *Consumer Reports* 2002; 67:26–31.

27. Jakicic JM, Clark K, Coleman E, Donnelly JE, Foreyt J, Melanson E, Volek J, Volpe SL; American College of Sports Medicine. American College of Sports Medicine position stand. Appropriate intervention strategies for weight loss and prevention of weight regain for adults. *Med Sci Sports Exerc.* 2001 Dec;33(12):2145–56.

28. Brehm BJ, Seeley RJ, Daniels SR, D'Alessio DA. A randomized trial comparing a very low carbohydrate diet and a calorie-restricted low fat diet on body weight and cardiovascular risk factors in healthy women. *J Clin Endocrinol Metab.* 2003 Apr;88(4):1617–23.

29. Bravata DM, Sanders L, Huang J, Krumholz HM, Olkin I, Gardner CD, Bravata DM. Efficacy and safety of low-carbohydrate diets: a systematic review. *JAMA.* 2003 Apr 9;289(14):1837–50.

30. Stern L, Iqbal N, Seshadri P, Chicano KL, Daily DA, McGrory J, Williams M, Gracely EJ, Samaha FF. The effects of low-carbohydrate versus conventional weight loss diets in severely obese adults: one-year follow-up of a randomized trial. *Ann Intern Med.* 2004 May 18;140(10):778–85.

31. Samaha FF, Iqbal N, Seshadri P, Chicano KL, Daily DA, McGrory J, Williams T, Williams M, Gracely EJ, Stern L. A low-carbohydrate as compared with a low-fat diet in severe obesity. *N Engl J Med.* 2003 May 22;348(21):2074–81.

32. Yancy WS Jr, Olsen MK, Guyton JR, Bakst RP, Westman EC. A low-carbohydrate, ketogenic diet versus a low-fat diet to treat obesity and hyperlipidemia: a randomized, controlled trial. *Ann Intern Med.* 2004 May 18;140(10):769–77.

33. Golay A, Allaz AF, Morel Y, de Tonnac N, Tankova S, Reaven G. Similar weight loss with low- or high-carbohydrate diets. *Am J Clin Nutr.* 1996 Feb;63(2):174–8.

34. Foster GD, Wyatt HR, Hill JO, McGuckin BG, Brill C, Mohammed BS, Szapary PO, Rader DJ, Edman JS, Klein S. A randomized trial of a low-carbohydrate diet for obesity. *N Engl J Med.* 2003 May 22;348(21):2082–90.

35. Atkins R. *Atkins for Life.* New York: St. Martin's Pr: 2003.

36. Pavlou KN, Krey S, Steffee WP. Exercise as an adjunct to weight loss and maintenance in moderately obese subjects. *Am J Clin Nutr.* 1989 May;49(5 Suppl):1115–23.

37. Sikand G, Kondo A, Foreyt JP, Jones PH, Gotto AM Jr. Two-year follow-up of patients treated with a very-low-calorie diet and exercise training. *J Am Diet Assoc.* 1988 Apr;88(4):487–8.

38. Wadden TA, Sternberg JA, Letizia KA, Stunkard AJ, Foster GD. Treatment of obesity by very low calorie diet, behavior therapy, and their combination: a five-year perspective. *Int J Obes.* 1989;13 Suppl 2:39–46.

39. Brownell KD. The central role of lifestyle change in long-term weight management. *Clin Cornerstone.* 1999;2(3):43–51.

Chapter 14

1. Grundy SM, Cleeman JI, Merz CN, Brewer HB Jr, Clark LT, Hunninghake DB, Pasternak RC, Smith SC Jr, Stone NJ; National Heart, Lung, and Blood Institute; American College of Cardiology Foundation; American Heart Association. Implications of recent clinical trials for the National Cholesterol Education Program Adult Treatment Panel III guidelines. *Circulation.* 2004 Jul 13;110(2):227–39.

2. McGuire HL, Svetkey LP, Harsha DW, Elmer PJ, Appel LJ, Ard JD. Comprehensive lifestyle modification and blood pressure control: a review of the PREMIER trial. *Clin Hypertens.* 2004 Jul;6(7):383–90.

3. Deen D. Metabolic syndrome: time for action. *Am Fam Physician.* 2004 Jun 15;69(12):2875–82.

4. Gerberding J. Director of the Centers for Disease Control and Prevention, Personal communication with the author, July 9, 2004.

5. Kaiser Family Foundation/Health Research and Educational Trust. Annual Employer Benefits Survey. Menlo Park (CA); 2003. Available online at www.kff.org/content/2003/20030909a/

6. U.S. Department of Health and Human Services, Public Health Service, 1992 National Survey of Worksite Health Promotion Activities: Summary, *Am J Health Promot.* 1993 7(6):452–464.

7. Wilson M, DeJoy D, Jorgensen C, Crump C. Health Promotion Programs in Small Worksites: Results of a National Survey. *Am J Health Promot.* 1999 13(6):358–365.

Useful Links on the Web

www.pubmed.gov
    Search for any health topic in the original research articles

www.hsph.harvard.edu/nutritionsource
    Harvard's great source for accurate nutrition information

www.cdc.gov/nccdphp/power_prevention/pdf/power_of_prevention.pdf
    The *Power of Prevention* brochure from the CDC

www.cfsan.fda.gov/label.html
    The USDA guide to reading nutrition labels

www.nutritiondata.com
    Find the nutrition labels for almost any food

www.glycemicindex.com
    Find the glycemic index for many foods

www.pedometer.com   www.pedometersusa.com
    Online sites to get good, inexpensive pedometers

www.HealthierUS.gov
>   The government's new program to promote healthy lifestyles

www.washoe.k12.nv.us/wellness
>   An example of a great worksite health-promotion program

www.ca-takeaction.com
>   Any worksite can offer its employees a great exercise program with this Web site

www.welcoa.org
>   Official Web site of the Wellness Councils of America that has a lot of great lifestyle change information and programs

www.nhlbi.nih.gov/health/public/heart/other/ktb_recipebk/
>   Healthy recipes from the National Institutes of Health

www.deliciousdecisions.org
>   Healthy recipes from the American Heart Association

www.fastfoodfacts.com
>   Order booklet containing nutritional information from most fast food restaurants

www.actionforhealthykids.org
>   Great ideas for helping children eat healthy and be active

www.butterfinger.com
>   An example of how marketing efforts makes it difficult to choose healthy foods

www.berkeleywellness.com
www.mayoclinic.com
www.health.harvard.edu/hhp/home.do
>   Accurate, unbiased sources of new health information

Recommended Books

Food Politics by Marion Nestle

5 a Day: The Better Health Cookbook by Elizabeth Pivonka

Quick & Healthy Recipes and Ideas: For People Who Say They Don't Have Time to Cook Healthy Meals by Brenda J. Ponichtera

Quick Meals for Healthy Kids and Busy Parents: Wholesome Family Recipes in 30 Minutes or Less from Three Leading Child Nutrition Experts by Sandra K. Nissenberg, Margaret L. Bogle, Audrey C. Wright

Healthy Treats and Super Snacks for Kids by Jeff MacNelly

Low-Fat Lies: High Fat Frauds & the Healthiest Diet in the World by Kevin Vigilante, Mary Flynn

Index

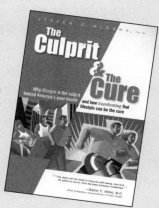